DEATH DOULA

TOOLS & TECHNIQUES FOR END-OF-LIFE SUPPORT

KELLY RUBY HANSON

Difference Press

Washington, DC, USA

Published 2021

DISCLAIMER

Cover design: Jennifer Stimson

Editing: Natasa Smirnov

Author's photo courtesy of: Cristina Julia

ADVANCE PRAISE

"*Death Doula* puts the silent and unacknowledged parts of the dying process into words. Opening the door for someone to gain a deeper understanding of the dying process. Giving knowledge to help the dying leave this earth with respect and grace. Taking you through the stages of death with a reverence for life and adding a bridge from the dying to the living."

— ASHLEY MCKENNA, LPCC, GRIEF AND LOSS THERAPIST

"The issue of death is beyond the personal. Concerning the individual, the book is an excellent guide on preparing for one's own departure as well as how to assist other people. What would it be like if people spent as much time and energy planning for their death as they do on planning for their wedding? Too many people I know think of death only in a medical context and not in a spiritual sense.

"This book is very well written and it is so needed!"

— FRANCES BLAINE

"Death has touched me closely several times in my life. I have lost both my parents in a hospital setting. My father died as a young man after an illness and my mother, later in life, very suddenly and unexpectedly. I believe these losses opened my heart at a young age to grief, to wondering about the mystery of death and to wondering if there are ways to prepare for it and support people as they move through their dying time in ways that feel more peaceful and open than what I experienced.

"*Death Doula* is the tender, honest, and thorough resource that I have been looking for about this topic. I now feel better prepared to have open and courageous conversations with my family about this topic. I especially loved Kelly Hanson's reminder that we can best support another person in their dying time by being present in our own life, by acknowledging our own range of emotions and by providing the kindness and compassion to ourselves that we hope to give to others as they are dying."

— VANESSA WOODBURN, CERTIFIED HEALTH COACH, EDUCATOR, AND AUTHOR OF *BOUNCE BACK: RECLAIM YOUR LIFE AFTER A CONCUSSION*

"As a how-to guide, this book contains everything you may need to know. It is brimming with straightforward strategies and vital information anyone can use to support people fully at the end of their life. This book will help our communities overcome the key fears associated with death and dying.

Anyone who's ever wanted to be able to confidently plan for a conscious, empowered, and gentle death can benefit from the down-to-earth knowledge in this book."

— JOANNA LINCOLNE, BIG LOVE CEREMONIES

"This book needs to be read by absolutely everybody. Kelly sheds light on a topic that so many of us shy away from. She is teaching us that death is a part of living that can be done with honour, integrity and compassion. She has captured the beauty of transitioning and showed us all that it is not to be feared. For anyone looking into death doula work, Kelly's experience and teachings will empower you in the most practical ways."

— LAURA DILL, CAREGIVING COACH AND AUTHOR OF *DAUGHTER: EMBRACING THE DIFFICULT JOURNEY OF CARING FOR A DYING PARENT WITHOUT FALLING APART*

"Wow, I truly wish I had the insights this book brings as I was in charge of the end-of-life process for a number of people important to my life two years ago. The deaths went well but could have been made better if I had a death doula available with the insightful and well thought out processes Kelly has created and shared through this wonderful and easy to read book."

— HEIDI THOMPSON-HENYON, AUTHOR,
ENERGY EDUCATOR, HEALTH COACH

CONTENTS

To my people...
To Reid for encouraging me to live life to its fullest.
To Terry for teaching me to see things differently.
And to Lilly for always telling me I should write a book.
I love you all.

1

DOING DEATH BETTER

No one ever told her about the little losses that come along with dying. They only ever mentioned the obvious – that her mother was dying. That is a big loss – one Betsy will mourn greatly – but there are so many other small changes that she does not think she is allowed to be sad over. She caught a glimpse of the almost daily losses years before when her grandfather went into the nursing home. He had always been such a big, strong man that took care of his family until he no longer could. Loss one was his strength. Loss two was his ability to live in his own home. Loss three was his memory. Until finally, he died. The biggest loss, her grandfather's death, was the one that most people gave condolences on, but his death did not just happen one day. It was as if his life was slowly chipped away at, and no one had language to help her cope with all of it.

Now, standing over her mother sleeping on the couch – noticing her swollen legs and her altered breathing – Betsy can see what no one around her is willing to talk about. Everything that makes up who her mother is is being slowly chipped away at. It is as though not talking about her mother's illness and impending death will somehow prevent it from happening. But she sees that her mom is struggling with not being allowed to talk about what she is losing. Her mom is losing her life in small increments. Daily, there are changes to the way she lives. Every time she wakes up, there is a new starting point for her body. The day before yesterday, she could breathe on her own. Today, she needs oxygen to help her breathe comfortably. Yesterday, she could get up and move around the house and interact with the people she lives with. Today, all she can do is sleep. She does not know if her mom is so tired because she is dying or if she is tired because no one is letting her die.

When her grandfather passed, Betsy saw firsthand how the people left behind could have a harder time grieving when they ignored the gradual changes he was experiencing. For her family, this meant that her grandfather's death came as a surprise when in fact the signs were clear the entire time that he was dying. Somewhere deep inside herself, Betsy began to realize that her grandfather's death could have been handled better, but she was not sure how.

It was not until later, when her mother got sick, that Betsy remembered the feelings she had during the end of her grandfather's life. Her mother's illness was much faster, and she had little time to do anything differently. She was at the mercy of her mom's disease, and when her mother died, Betsy felt relief, sadness, and anger. Betsy wanted to talk to her mother about the fact that she was dying but did not know where to start. Her mother was in her sixties, and she seemed too young to die. Betsy didn't know where to begin the conversation with her mom. It felt too difficult a talk. She saw the swift changes in her mom's body and her ability to function, but no one had the language to talk about how she was losing pieces of her mom every day. Her mom's death was the final loss, but her heart had already endured so much hurt watching her mom die. These little losses remained unacknowledged and unprocessed, and as such, they were amplifying Betsy's pain.

What Betsy experienced is not uncommon. When faced with the idea of someone in our lives dying, we have little idea of how to handle the situation, what to say to each other, and especially what to say to the dying person. We do not know how to make room for the little losses and the tough and unsolicited changes that we must accept. We have not been taught how to approach the subject of death, which is ironic since, as humans, we will all one day die.

So, what are we taught about death and dying? The subject of death is closeted away. It is brought out only in small doses, and it is even taboo to speak of the little losses that happen during the dying process when we are with someone who is actually dying. Hiding the reality of death only makes living the experience more difficult for the dying person and the people surrounding them. It seems like we have a well-rehearsed script to use when talking about death. This script includes what happened in a person's life before they learned that they were dying, and then it jumps to the grief that ensues after death occurs. But we are not allowed to talk about the process in between. See, between living and death lies a whole host of experiences that are begging to be acknowledged and supported. The gap between dying and being dead is where the skills of a death doula are best utilized.

Not many people are comfortable talking about the dying experience. For many, death is just something that happens. Those left behind move on. If they have trouble moving on, they do not talk about it. As Betsy started to realize, we can handle the time between dying and being dead better. A person's dying time can be a time for healing, growth, and acceptance. And for some, that healing can come long after the deaths have occurred, like for Betsy.

In our work together, Betsy was able to review her mom's and her grandfather's dying experiences and identify what would have better helped her at the time. She was also able to develop a better understanding of how those experiences were still impacting her – mainly, how those two difficult events could make her want to grow and help someone else when faced with their death live fully during the little time they have left. It was these insights and Betsy's innate compassion and empathy that propelled her decision to become a death doula.

Betsy's curiosity about working with those in the dying process started her on the path of working with me to better understand the emotional loads she carried concerning the deaths and grief surrounding the many losses that went unsupported when her loved ones were dying. She felt called to serve more than just the symptoms a dying person experiences. She wanted to bring sacredness to the dying process by learning to support the person as a whole. More importantly, by training with me to become a death doula, Betsy not only learned how to support others, but she also began to heal herself.

Does Betsy's story resonate with you? Do you hear your heart timidly whispering that there is a better way to handle death? There most certainly is, and you've come to the right place. In this book, I am going to help you hear that intrinsic wisdom more clearly and teach you the sacred ways of end-of-life doulas. Let's demystify the dying process to bring much-needed healing to yourself and others with a conscious, communal, and authentic approach to the complex end-of-life processes. I hear you. I see you. And I can help.

2

HOW I BECAME A DEATH DOULA

It started with one question. "Will you be okay without me?" my mother asked. Pushing down tears, I told her, "No, I will not be okay." I asked her if she would be okay. I didn't know if her response was for me or her. "I'll be okay. I'll be okay."

But she wasn't. My mom was diagnosed with lung cancer in the spring of 2013. She was gone by Friday, May 31st, the same year. The time between her diagnosis and her death moved differently for me. It was fast and slow at the same time. When my mom asked me if I would be okay after she was gone, I was working my normal weekend night shift at the hospital. Thankfully, it was a calm season, and there were not many deaths. It was not always that way. I worked in the operating room. Most of my twenty years in healthcare were spent working off shifts at level-one trauma hospitals. My surgical training had taught me that I could deal with intense and complicated procedures and patient circumstances. Sherri Alexander, my clinical educator put it more plainly when she told my class, "Sometimes patients come to you already dead." While that may sound harsh or cold to you, it was helpful for me because of her explanation. She stood before a room of newly trained healthcare professionals and told us the truth. Some of us would go to work at facilities that treated patients that came in so badly injured, so past help, that it would be our job to do everything that we could to save these people. But we would not be able to save everyone no matter how hard we tried. I cannot say for certain if my classmates lived Sherri's words. I did; even before I graduated.

During one of the hardest weekends in my early career, we lost nine patients. But that was not my first exposure to death. By that point in my life, I had lost three of my grandparents, an aunt, two friends, several pets, and several older more distant family members. My mom never shied away from talking about her opinions on medical choices with me when I was a teenager, and my parents never hid death or severe illness from me. Even at my first job waiting tables, it seemed as though the world was preparing me to work with ill and dying people. My server job was at a small country restaurant where many of the opening customers were elderly who did not seem to have much family around them. The family they did have had either moved away or did not come around to visit. My coworker, a woman my own mother's age, taught me to pay attention to all the customers and to get to know them as if we were close friends or family. Many of our customers came in every day at the same time. She taught me to pay especially close attention to the ones who seemed to be on their own. We would call them at home if they did not show up at the restaurant. We would talk with them about their health and their lives. We had memorized their favorite foods and knew how to adjust it if their stomachs were upset or their teeth hurt. It was during this time that I learned to watch for a surge in energy in those people who were close to dying. All this I learned from listening to my coworker and by watching our older customers. It was a good learning experience.

In college, there was a course called "Death and Dying" in the psychology department. I heard from other students that it was a class that I needed to take. "It's life-changing." I did not take this class. Instead, I lived the class. Maybe if I had taken the class, I would have had an easier time dealing with all the loss I encountered in my personal life and all the death I would face in my career. Like I said, I did not take the class, but I would take many classes and read many books later in life that covered what was probably taught in the class.

I cannot say for certain, but my time spent in the operating room seemed to be filled with more death than the people in my same position seemed to experience. I cannot even begin to count on my hands and feet the number of bodies I have cleaned up and put into body bags. I guess it went with the hours I worked (weekends and weekend nights) and the type of hospitals (level-one trauma hospitals) I worked at. More importantly, like my time waiting tables, I learned to watch and listen to the nurses who had more experience with losing patients. I learned how to make a patient look warm and comfy in a hospital bed while hiding the body bag under the blankets. I learned to thoroughly clean the deceased's hands because they would often be held by their loved ones. I also learned not to ignore the immensity of witnessing someone's end of life. The hospital did not provide any services for those teams that had lost patients. The exception was if the loss was traumatic for the team. I found this funny because, in my experience, every loss – no matter how expected – was hard to go through, and those facing it could benefit from support.

I began to learn to find my own way of dealing with the intensity of my work. Once again, my coworkers were invaluable resources. Many times in my career, I found myself being with the families of the patient we lost. It is not normal for a surgical tech to inform a daughter that her mother had died or to sit with a family as they take time after a person's passing. What made it more difficult and more beautiful was that I was also on the team working to save the patient's life. I did chest compressions, held pressure on bleeding wounds, and then had to help clean the patient up and get them ready for their family. These experiences were difficult and beautiful in that while spending time with the remaining family members, I got to learn about the patient we had fought so hard for. I got to know them a little.

In all the losses I have experienced, there usually came a point in time when I would look up at the sky or ceiling and think, maybe even ask the universe, "Why is this happening? Why can't we do this better?" I had seen in my own family both how a person can die a good death and a bad one. Often, the factor determining the difference between the two was having conversations with people about the person's wishes and not actively fighting the fact that person was dying. I am all for advanced medical care and trying sometimes aggressive forms of treatment, but I also have felt it in my heart and soul that sometimes we take it too far. Death is 100 percent fatal for 100 percent of people. I wondered how I could begin to work to support people to understand this and not run away from it as a society.

It was clear to me very early on in my healthcare career that many people did not want to "sit and talk about death" with me. Even terminally ill people were hesitant. So, that led me to take my medical knowledge, my lived experiences, my education and training, and begin to work as a death doula.

Someone once told me that I became a death doula to find a way to cope with losing my mom. I said that was absolutely true, and why shouldn't it be? Why must we act like death and grief are something that can be neatly packaged up and processed quickly? Why can't death be something that we can learn about and strive to do better long before our own dying time? I noticed something was missing inside myself, and I wanted to fill that gap with knowledge and better understanding of how to be with the dying for their sake and my own. What I originally sought out to console my own heart and experiences became a gift that I have been able to share with others. I help people who are trying to cope with a cherished person's dying process. I also support people who are deep in grief, as well as healthy individuals far from death who want to ensure their people are cared for and their wishes met when they do die. I guide people going through the physical, emotional, and spiritual process of dying. My work as a death doula is a culmination of my skills as an observer of others' experiences, my ability to build a safe container to allow for a full range of emotions, and my willingness to be with people as they move through a trying time.

I believe this work to be essential. More importantly, it's healing work. I am, therefore, committed to teaching others to do it. Death is something that we all face. We all live mortal lives that will one day end. If things work out as they should, older family members or friends who have had the chance to live full lives will die before us and we will learn from them. Even when that happens, those loved ones deserve more layers of support and so do the people surrounding them. Being supported in their dying time serves the dying, but indirectly, it shows us how dying can be lived more fully.

Death and dying encompass so much that is unknown to us. Even the parts that we do understand can be scary. Supporting people during the dying process asks much of an individual. It asks everything of the dying person, and it takes much from those surrounding them. Yes, it is an honor and gift when someone trusts you enough to be with them during their dying time or to talk openly about their experience, but that gift also lies in the shadow of a burden – the burden of what you have to see and experience when you sit with the dying. It is the burden of facing your own mortality. To be a death doula, a person must firmly look mortality in the face while continuing to be present in their own lives. This is why it is important to train more people in the art of being a death doula. Whether they end up working as a doula, volunteering, or being a doula for a loved one does not matter. What is asked of the individual supporting the dying can break them if unprepared. But it can also heal them. Dying and death are not straightforward experiences. There are many nuances that people should learn in order to be a well-versed death doula.

My desire to create a program to train death doulas comes from the same place as my desire to teach new surgical technologists to work on the team of some of the most difficult surgeries. Put simply, I see that people can do hard things when they are supported and taught in a way that makes them feel safe. Not to brag, but I am going to brag... The majority of surgical technologists that I precepted in my career went on to work on some of the most stressful teams and support the most challenging surgeries. They learned to endure tough procedures where the patients were very ill and the surgeons were not always nice. Their confidence started developing when I gave them the steps of what was going to take place, what their part in all of it was, and how I was going to support them. Those are the same things you will find in this book.

By reading this book, you are showing that you have in you a gift and a strength that means you can do this work. And that you will be good at it. Even if you only perform the duties of a death doula one time or a hundred times or not at all, learning these skills will empower you to live more fully while supporting others, whatever that looks like. This book will teach you that you can do difficult things. I am here to support you as you begin to embody that idea. So, buckle up. There is a lot to cover.

3

THE PATH TO BECOMING A DEATH DOULA

"It is for everyone, for all people, young and old, rich and poor, religious or not, should give attention to the art of dying well by living well throughout their lives."

— L.S. DUGDALE

Once I started claiming the title death doula in my work, the response I would often get was, "Oh, that is so needed... So, what is it that you do?" How could people state that my work was so needed and in the same breath ask for clarification on what it involves? Easily.

The job death doula is a relatively new field of work, and not many people understand what services they provide. What people have grown aware of is that there is a disconnect between what people say they want at their dying time and what takes place. Death doulas bridge this gap with their doula bags and unique set of skills and talents.

While the work of caring for the dying is not new, the unique ability of a death doula to blend ancient ways of being present for another person with modern practices ensures personalized, nonjudgmental care that promotes personal growth and agency for those they serve.

Our current model of care for the dying does not facilitate caring for the dying person in a holistic way. Much of the work done in our Western medical model is focused on treating the physical diminishment of the body and forestalling death. Medical professionals and family members provide much in the way of care when it comes to supporting someone at the end of their life. Do not get me wrong, people who work with the dying in the Western medical model of care are amazing and their work is necessary, but there is room for improvement. There is room for caring for the dying in a holistic way that takes into consideration that a person is more than their body and that death is more than a medical and religious experience.

SO, YOU WANT TO BE A DEATH DOULA?

Now that you have decided to become a death doula, do you really know what that means? If you were like me and those who have commented on my work, you know it is essential, but you are not 100 percent sure about what the work entails. Maybe you feel called to do this work as Betsy did because of her life experiences and maybe you already work with ill and dying populations and want to deepen your connections with them. Whatever the reason may be that you were called to this work, you are already on track to be an effective death doula by reading this book. Your curiosity and desire to do things better, to do them differently is what brought you here. Now, let's cover what is essential to learn in order to best serve your clients, your family members, and the world at large because we are all connected. If we can work to ensure that everyone has the opportunity to die a good death, then we will all benefit. By learning and developing better ways to communicate about and share in the dying process, we will grow in our ability to live. We will grow in our acceptance of life's limits, we will cherish our abilities and relationships, and we will become more open to life's possibilities.

This book will cover tools and techniques that will allow you to support someone in their dying time as a death doula.

The chapters will guide you through the following topics:

- Physical changes that occur and medical language used during the dying process.

- How different emotions and behaviors can affect the dying process and what that means for the death doula.

- How to create a deathbed environment based on someone's wishes and values by using advanced communications techniques.

- Hands-on techniques for supporting a dying person.

- Importance of rituals in supporting the dying, accessible examples of rituals, and how to create new ones.

- Owning and embodying being a death doula

- Walking through the steps of building an end-of-life plan with you as your first client.

Throughout the chapters, you will find sections called *Death Doula Starter Pack*. The questions in the sections are meant to develop your understanding of your personal being and what your relationship is to death. Additionally, you will find questions that can be used with your clients in this section. They are meant to be used to spark deep conversations while aiding in end-of-life planning by accessing deep, sometimes hard-to-reach places in your client's soul and life experiences. In the Death Doula Starter Pack sections, you will also find specific exercises that allow you to put your work into action.

The reflections, exercises, and client questions in the Death Doula Starter Pack sections of the book are set up for you to walk through them as you read the book. They are also designed so that you can return to them at any point in time in your practice of being a death doula. There may be parts of the book that covers information that you are already familiar with. Great! Save yourself some time, and skim over those parts. There also may be parts of the book that make you feel uncomfortable. If that is the case, give yourself some grace and come back to those parts when you feel more ready. Not all the tools and techniques covered in this book will be used by every person. All the information in this book was chosen based on what I believe will best teach people to be well-rounded death doulas. That means there is a lot of information presented in this book. That does not mean you have to memorize it. What information, tools, and techniques you implement from this book will depend on where you serve dying people and what offerings you provide to them.

My style of teaching someone to be a death doula extends from my days of precepting or training people to work in the operating room. I break down the art of being a death doula into the components and focus on developing critical thinking skills that will serve you in any deathbed space you enter. In the operating room, much to the dismay of the people I was training, my favorite phrases when asked questions included "It depends" and "What do you think?" Those responses are still my most frequently used answers to questions because a person's ability to work as a death doula relies on their critical thinking skills and their ability to be flexible in their actions in different situations while relying on foundational knowledge in the area of death and dying. Working with dying people means working in a realm with few clear-cut answers. This book is filled with foundational information along with questions to ask yourself and your clients to develop your doula skills and the idea that in order to serve dying people, first, we must face our own mortality.

So now, allow yourself to see fully the sacredness that presents itself during the dying process and the beauty of the heart-to-heart connections you will form with the people you serve. After all, even when a person is dying, they are still living.

4

THE PHYSICAL PARTS OF DYING

The medicalization and closeting away of death limited many people's exposure to dying. And when you do experience death, it seems like understanding it is reserved solely for the professionals providing medical care or after-death services. Even those of us who have worked in healthcare may not have the language to explain to the family or the patient's people what is happening. Sometimes, we do not have the courage to point out the physical changes occurring and state that this is what dying looks like. It is human to avoid causing hurt and to want to shield those surrounding a dying person. The prospect of losing a loved one can be scary. But keeping the process hidden away and not discussing it fuels this fear. We fear what we do not understand. Knowledge and information can be key to reducing fear when it comes to dying.

As death doulas, we have to allow space for family members who may not want the information, but as supporters of the process, we must be well-versed in the physical components of dying. Your work with the dying will position you to have an awareness of what could happen, but you will not always have all the answers, and you will not be able to guarantee exactly what will take place. Having an understanding of the physical plane of dying will build your knowledge base, increase your ability to speak the language of death, and give you a measure of confidence needed to walk into a room where you know you are supporting someone in death. This chapter will cover topics such as:

- Pre-active and active stages of dying
- Breathing changes
- Skin changes
- Temperature changes
- Changes in activity levels
- Sleep changes and disturbances
- Other physical signs of dying
- Physical signs that death has occurred

Instead of memorizing the physical signs of the human body transitioning through the dying process, you can reference your own body. If you are reading this book, then you have a body. No matter your physical condition, your ableness, your level of health, your own body can provide a point of reference when interacting with other people to get a better understanding of what they are experiencing. I was taught to do this when training for surgery. Anytime I needed to figure out how to position a patient for procedures or what area of the body we were going to be working on, my teacher would stop me and ask me to show them on my own body if I was having trouble visualizing the answers. We often worked together on traumatic bone injuries that had many complications. Before the surgery, we would talk about how to position the patient and what supplies we would need. To communicate his ideas to me, the doctor would grab my arm or my leg and talk through his thoughts while moving my limb into the position he would want the patient's in. He would also point out where on my extremity the injury was. By allowing the surgeon to reference my own physical being, I was able to integrate better how and why we chose options to treat a patient over others and the reasons behind those choices. It strengthened my critical thinking, and I learned to own that way of thinking in my body. One goal of this section is to develop those same skills in you.

There is no right or wrong way for a person to live through their dying process, and the following physical aspects of dying may or may not present in every person. Dying does follow a general pattern with some specific signs indicating the end is near, but death is experienced in its own way by every individual. Much like a person labors to birth a child, a person must labor in the dying process. It requires effort to die.

The rhythm of dying can be explained in physical stages otherwise known as symptoms. Sometimes stages or symptoms may be lingered in or completely passed over. The physical aspects we will cover pertain to gradual death, not traumatic deaths or abrupt unexpected deaths.

WHEN DEATH IS NEAR

The physical plane of dying involves the body's shut-down processes. It is a normal part of preparing to stop living. One thing to note is that dying is often not painful. Pain usually comes from previous disease processes, treatments, or positioning of the body. The physical plane of dying is made up of stages called pre-active and active dying. The pre-active stage is the time leading up to the active labor of death. Pre-active dying can last around three weeks and typically shows up as increased mental and physical restlessness and withdrawal from active participation in life, along with increased periods of sleep. There may also be increased changes to the person's physical appearance. It is even possible that no signs will present at all during this stage. Active dying is the final stage of the dying process. It can last as few as three days, but the timeline for active death can be different depending on the dying person. The actively dying person is very near to death and may show signs such as being unresponsive and having a significant drop in blood pressure. Factors that can impact how a person transitions through the phases include types of illnesses they are experiencing, types of medical treatments received, and the quality of the individual's care.

Pre-active dying signs and symptoms are:

- Increased restlessness, confusion, agitation, inability to stay content in one position, and insisting on changing positions frequently (exhausting family and caregivers)

- Withdrawal from active participation in social activities

- Increased periods of sleep, lethargy

- Decreased intake of food and liquids

- Beginning to show periods of pausing in the breathing (apnea) whether awake or sleeping

- Visions of persons who have already died

- Person states that he or she is dying

- Person requests family visit to settle "unfinished business" and tie up "loose ends"

- Inability to heal or recover from wounds or infections

- Increased swelling (edema) of either the extremities or the entire body

- Active dying stage signs include:

- Inability to swallow any fluids at all (not taking any food by mouth voluntarily as well)

- Person states that he or she is going to die

- Breathing through wide-open mouth continuously and no longer can speak even if awake

- Urinary or bowel incontinence in a person who was not incontinent before

- Marked decrease in urine output and darkening color of urine or very abnormal colors (such as red or brown)

- Blood pressure dropping dramatically from person's normal blood pressure range (more than a twenty- or thirty-point drop; systolic blood pressure below 70, diastolic blood pressure below 50)

• Extremities (such as hands, arms, feet, and legs) feel very cold to touch

• Complaints that legs/ feet are numb and cannot be felt at all

• Cyanosis, or a bluish or purple coloring to the person's arms and legs, especially the feet and hands

• Body remains in rigid, unchanging position

• Jaw drop; the patient's jaw is no longer held straight and may drop to the side, their head lying toward

What is important during the active dying phase is to be present with the person, provide comfort care, facilitate positive interactions with the people around them. It is not the time to focus on curative medical interventions. It is not a time to fix things. Our current model of medical care focuses on fixing things – illnesses, injuries, and even death. While that model of care is not completely wrong, it does provide a false sense to people that death can be avoided at all costs.

Our current model of medical care also has established ranges for what "normal" looks like for people – a picture of what health looks like that does not make space for many people in our society. A death doula can be flexible in their idea of "normal" and be open to a wider range of what is normal based on the person in front of them instead of relying solely on the medical model. Doulas are not there to judge or measure health ranges or lifestyle choices. A death doula is there to see the person as they are, for who they are, and to best support them as their new normal changes daily throughout the dying process. Regardless of a person's level of ableness, their race, religion, ailments, we are there to support them – sometimes when there is no one else willing to do so.

Being comfortable with the signs and symptoms of the phases of death will allow you – the death doula – to properly support the dying person's circle by being able to explain what your client is experiencing. It will also empower you to help your client relax into their experience as stress and pain can prolong the dying process.

Breathing

One of the most visible signs during the dying process is the changes in breathing patterns. While this can be distressing to witness, these changes are often not uncomfortable for the person. If discomfort is experienced, alert the hospice team or managing physician in order for them to order medications that will provide comfort care without extending life. This can include the use of morphine or supplemental oxygen.

The changes in breathing patterns can include irregular breathing which means the time between breaths can stretch out with many seconds or even minutes. The person can also take several breaths in succession and have a long pause before their breathing resumes. This is referred to as Cheyne-Stokes breathing. Apnea is another term used in relation to breathing, and it is the absence of breathing. Dying people can have periods of apnea and resume a normal breathing pattern.

Breathing can also become louder. The dying person may not be able to swallow or cough which can lead to a gurgling sound or the "death rattle." This does not cause pain for the person but can be difficult to hear for those around the bedside. Doctors comment about how relaxed the person is that they do not care about the secretions that build up. "Fish-out-of-water" breathing can also be observed. This occurs when a person gasps for air.

Skin Changes

Skin changes that occur during the dying process are usually due to the reduced circulation of oxygen-carrying blood throughout the body. Skin color changes also happen due to the kidneys slowing down. This can result in a person's skin appearing a different color such as purplish, pale grey, yellowish (different than jaundice coloring), or bluish (cyanosis). The skin can also become blotchy or mottled, especially on the hands, feet, and knees. The person's fingertips can especially show signs of circulation decreases. With a gentle squeeze on someone's fingertip, their nail bed can show signs of how fast their capillary response is. Push on your fingertip right now with your other hand and watch how quickly it goes from whitish back to its regular color. A person's normal skin color can affect how the skin color changes present.

The dying person's ability to feel sensations on their arms and legs may decrease. They may feel numb. The arms and legs may also show signs of swelling (edema) and the body is no longer moving fluid around as it does in regular circumstances. Swelling can also present in the entire body. Because the dying person is experiencing reduced circulation, they will also have an impaired ability to heal from wounds.

Skin changes also may be affected by any diseases the person has such as diabetes or heart disease. Some of the skin changes that occur in the dying body also show up in different disease processes. It is important to be aware of what symptoms a person has in their daily life to establish what their normal skin condition is and how any changes show up in their body during their transition.

Temperature

A person in their dying journey can experience a wide range of temperature fluctuations. It is common for people to express that they are cold, and their hands can feel cold to the touch. It is also not uncommon for someone to feel overheated. Temperature is important to pay attention to because it can affect how the dying person acts. A person who is overheated can become agitated and restless. A person who is cold can move less and feel stiffer. Both can affect pain tolerance for different reasons. Metabolic changes that the person experiences can also lead to clamminess and excessive perspiration or sweating.

Output

As the body functions slow down, the kidneys gradually slow or stop producing urine. This can also be related to a decrease in fluid intake. This slowing and/ or stopping can cause urine to become darker in color, often brown or dark red. Changes in bowel movements can also take place. If a person is on narcotics to assist in pain management, then constipation is likely to occur. Again, constipation can also be present due to decreased fluid intake.

Many people express concern over losing control of their bladder and bowels. This is a possibility, but it does not happen to everyone. As a practicing death doula, you will learn to be discrete when speaking about this topic and identify quickly who is willing to talk about it and help with cleaning up urine and bowel movements. This can be managed by hospice staff or paid caregivers, but often informal caregivers and family members take care of cleaning up after a dying person. It is important to maintain a high level of hygiene when it comes to urination and stool. Not only can sitting in urine or stool negatively impact a person's skin condition, but it also affects their dignity.

Sleep

Sleep is a common sign in both the pre-active dying stage and the active dying stage. In both cases, the sleep can be more like a coma where the person cannot easily be roused. This is normal, and the person should be allowed to rest. It will not be necessary to wake someone to give them fluids or food. Depending on the situation, it may be important to wake someone to administer pain medication. This is usually at the discretion of the physician in charge of the person's care or the hospice team. Waking a person for pain medication will help maintain a better level of pain control, which is essential for the person's relaxation. If the body is not relaxed, then it can fight the process of dying.

It is also possible for a person to experience insomnia during their dying journey. Comfort care can be provided by the medical team to aid a person in this area.

Mental Confusion

It is common for dying people to experience confusion. This can be due to many reasons, some medical and some spiritual. People can have illusions where they misperceive objects in their room. It is a misunderstanding of something that is actually in their surroundings.

Hallucinations are also common. Dying people can hear voices, see things that are not there, and feel things. Some people can experience delusions. They can think that the people who are caring for them are trying to harm them. They can also begin to think that they can accomplish anything.

Identifying confusion or abnormal mental behaviors is more easily done with reference points. If you have had a relationship prior to the person entering the later phases of the dying process, it is helpful because you know the person better and will have an idea of what normal looks like for them. If this has not happened, it is okay. As death doulas, we must accept the idea that everyone starts off with different levels of mental capacities. Collecting information on and understanding any prior mental diagnoses may help, but you may not have access to this information. Often this change is harder to go through for family members and people close to the dying person than it is for those attending the bedside. The death doula's reassurance that these changes are normal and that the person is still there even though their behavior may be different will bring a world of comfort to those surrounding the person.

Food and Fluid Intake

Journeying through the dying process takes energy, both physical and spiritual or inner world energy. In normal life, we receive our energy through the food we eat and the liquids we drink. While there will be times that the dying person's energy will need to be replenished with food and drink, there will come a time when those things are no longer needed. It will be as though the person will be fueled by something else, something intangible. Eating and drinking also may become difficult if the person begins to struggle with swallowing. It is important to not feed or give liquids to a person that is not awake or that is having difficulty swallowing, as this can lead to choking.

Speaking Less

There can be a time after a doctor has informed someone that there is nothing more than can be done for them or that they have a terminal illness when the person begins to turn inward. The desire to participate in the world with words diminishes, and they turn their focus inward. This can be due to a decrease in physical energy, mental cloudiness or brain fog, or lack of desire.

Moving Less

As a person's body prepares for death by slowly decreasing its functions, the dying person can begin to move less. This can also be due to pain or temperature discomfort that can be helped with comfort care measures. Another body positioning change that can occur is jaw drop. Jaw drop is when the person's jaw or chin does not stay straight. Instead, it may drop to the side that their head is lying as they are no longer able to hold their head straight. It is as though the jaw becomes loose.

This is an area where it helps to have a relationship with the person prior to their deathbed so you can have developed an understanding of what the person's normal is. People have varying levels of activity in life, different physical abilities, some have pre-existing conditions that affect how well and how often they move. It will be important to reference their normal baseline and not your own body or life experience here. What the dying person's normal looks like can change daily. It is your job to be fluid and work to identify changes in movement to make sense of what it means.

Terminal Restlessness

Another change that can manifest in the dying body is what is termed terminal restlessness. Restlessness occurs when the person cannot relax or rest. The person can show signs of agitation due to physical, emotional, or mental unrest. Dying can be a time of emotional and mental upheaval, which can be challenging for the person experiencing it to go through. The high levels of agitation can be caused by physiological changes such as metabolic failure causing organ failure which can interfere with brain function. Terminal restlessness can also be due to medications or poor pain management. It shows up in the dying person as wandering attention, outburst, aimlessness, or behaviors that do not match regular personality and appear suddenly.

Blood Pressure, Circulation, and Reduced Metabolic Function

Changes in the body's ability to move blood throughout the body will affect all areas of the person's physical being. Effects can be seen in skin changes, breathing patterns, blood pressure, pulse (heart beats per minute), energy levels, increases in sleeping, decreases in sleeping… basically everything. It affects what we can see and what we can't see. These changes are normal. Any treatments of this area should be focused on providing comfort, easing symptoms, and not fixing the reasons behind the reduced function. It is good to have an awareness of what normal ranges are, even as a nonmedical supporter of the dying. (Normal blood pressure according to the American Heart Association is 120/ 80. Normal pulse rate is 60-100 beats per minute. Normal respiration rate 12-16 breaths per minute.) The reason to know the normal ranges is to help you as their death doula track where your client is in the dying process. It is not necessary to have these ranges memorized. Remember, you are going to be referencing your own body when interacting with the people you are supporting. The ability to do this is based on the idea that you are aware of your health, your baseline for normal functions, and pay attention to the information that the medical team is collecting when you are with your health provider. Think back to an appointment when someone, maybe a medical assistant, was taking your blood pressure and your pulse. They should tell you those numbers, at least your blood pressure. If you were calm, then the numbers were probably your normal resting blood pressure and resting heart rate. If you were feeling anxious about the appointment, then those numbers could have been elevated. Even if the numbers were not spoken, recall how you felt. Was your heart beating hard and fast like you had been walking upstairs? Or was it not very noticeable like how it is when you are watching a calm show on Netflix? The idea of this exercise is not to recall the specific numbers or exact reason for your increase or decrease in blood pressure or pulse, but to start to identify a non-medical way of describing and identifying the experience within yourself. Working on this skill will benefit you in your own life as you become more accustomed to the physical language of your own body while it strengthens your skill in communicating with those that you are aiding in their time of transition. It is very common to have people talk about these physical aspects in nonmedical terms.

DEPRESSION AND ANXIETY

It is common for someone who is dying to experience anxiety and depression. Consider all that the person is facing. It makes sense for a person to feel sad when they know their life is ending. It also makes sense to be anxious because of all the unknown factors that are involved. Many times, people will end up on medications to treat these issues. While they can be helpful, medications may not be necessary if the dying person is receiving proper support. Also, accepting the fact that a person who is in their dying time has the right to feel anxious and depressed about their situation can help them have moments when they do not feel those emotions. A dying person may be facing the fact that their life plans did not turn out as they wanted or making peace with the choices that they should not have made. They may also be coming to terms with all the hardships that they had to face in their life. There is also the physical diminishment that they experience.

A dying person deserves the right to have a full range of emotions concerning what they are experiencing. If they desire to take medication to help with depression or anxiety, then they should have it, but they should also be provided with adequate mental and emotional support in other forms. By not allowing someone to be sad or nervous about their dying time, it in effect can alienate the person and make their dying time a lonely experience.

THE SURGE/ SUNSET DAY

A sunset day, also known as a surge day, is a period of time when a person in the dying process may suddenly experience moments of increased strength, heightened lucidity or increased mental clarity, and have more energy. It is as though they experience a surge of strength to accomplish the next part of their dying process, their actual death. It is also not unusual for the dying person to request favorite foods or drinks during this time. This usually occurs a few days before a person dies. It can be a good time for the circle of people surrounding the dying person to have healing conversations or to create cherished memories.

AFTER DEATH

So, what does death look like? The labor of death can vary in the amount of time it takes and can pass over certain stages and linger in others. Complicated emotions can arise at this time, as a dying person's labor requires not only effort from them but also those surrounding them. Although every person's death is unique and personal to them, there are general signs that can be looked for to know that death has occurred. These include:

- Breathing stops
- No heartbeat or pulse felt
- Person cannot be woken up
- Eyelids may be half-open
- Mouth may remain open
- Pupils are fixed

The after-death process does not need to be rushed. The timeline will of course depend on what facility the person has died in and the staff's willingness to allow people time with their loved one, whether it be at home, a hospital, or a nursing facility. As the practicing death doula, you can advocate for more time and protect the circle around the deceased.

Once death has occurred, no one has to be contacted

immediately if the person died at home. If the death happened at night, then contacting the primary physician managing the care of the person or the hospice staff can wait until morning. Follow the different state/ county/ province protocols for reporting death. Take time to educate yourself on what the local laws are concerning who to report the death to, who can confirm the death, and how long a body can stay at home. If hospice has been supporting the dying person, then they will be the primary resource for this information.

Medically, there are two stages of death. The first is clinical death, and it is when a person's heart stops beating. Breathing will stop, as will any movements. The second stage is biological death. It occurs four to six minutes after a person's heart stops beating. Brain cells will begin to die from lack of oxygen at this point. Knowing this is key in preventing any unwanted resuscitation attempts. Resuscitation can be successful during the clinical death stage. If emergency services or 911 is called and arrives at this stage, the paramedics and EMTs will work to resuscitate unless the proper paperwork, a do-not-resuscitate order (DNR), has been completed and is present.

Not moving the deceased from their deathbed can provide an opportunity for friends and relatives to come and say goodbye. Promptly removing the body and rushing the decedent's people along can have negative effects on their ability to grieve.

It is a good idea to make sure the room remains cool by removing any heat sources (lower thermostat if it has been set high, remove free-standing heaters, turn off electric blankets, remove any hot water bottles). The decedent's body will begin to stiffen, so straighten the person's limbs and position arms across the body. Take the time to replace dentures that were removed if it is what they wanted. There are further preparations that will need to be made if the decedent wants a home funeral or there are plans for extending the time before the body is removed. Chapter 9 will cover this in more detail along with options for rituals and body care ceremonies that can take place at this time.

DEATH DOULA STARTER PACK

Has anyone important in your life died?
Have you experienced a death in person?
Have you touched a dead body?
What types of end-of-life ceremonies have you experienced?

5

THE UNKNOWN – EVERYTHING BUT THE BODY

"When we talk about the importance of death, it's really essential for us to realize that death is something that we can and should become acquainted with before we die."

— CANDICE O'DENVER

What does Candice mean by "get acquainted with death"? We can familiarize ourselves with the physical goings-on with the body during the dying process, but anybody who attended someone at the bedside knows that there is more to the process than the events and changes that take place in the body. The fragility of the physical self and the disconnection from the everyday hustle and bustle of life strip away a person's ability to hide behind their job titles, their wealth, their status, and whatever else attachments they had to the material world. It is then that some people openly reflect on their lives, although not necessarily out loud. With this stripping away of the protective layers, the mysteries surrounding life and death become more visible, not just for the dying person, but also for those who are at their bedside.

We must give way to our certainty and allow space for the shifts, the unknown, and the unexplainable that take place during the human experience of death.

SLOW DOWN

> *"Give your certainty about things a rest for the duration and allow your wandering muscle a little exercise."*
>
> — STEPHEN JENKINSON

There is scientific evidence that our perception of time can be influenced by our emotions and the activity we are engaging in. The way we feel plays an integral role in how we experience the passing of seconds and minutes. Time perception is not a tangible attribute like our other senses and what we perceive. Our ability to feel motion, to hear sound, and to see objects seems concrete. Spend any time with a dying person and you will notice that the passage of time seems to change. Whether you are at the person's bedside or far away, once a terminal diagnosis is received or the body starts to shut down due to old age, it is as though time slows down. Days seem like weeks. Weeks like months. Even more confusing is that along with time slowing down, it also feels as though it's speeding up. There is not enough time to say all the words that need to be said or do all the things left undone. It is as though people become suspended in a sort of time limbo and nothing can be done about it. There is no medication or direct treatment for extensional change in perception of time. It must be endured by both those supporting the dying and by the person themselves. Dr.

Sarah Kerr, death doula, ritual practitioner, and a long-time student of cross-cultural healing and nature-based spirituality, teaches about soul time and what it means in her Ritual Skills for Living and Dying courses. Sarah explains that the outer being's time is not matched with what occurs for the inner being or the soul. She suggests that our souls need time to catch up with what is happening, especially in a person's dying time. Our inner being is not able to process the external and material changes that occur during dying as quickly as needed because Western culture is not practiced in investing in our inner selves in a way that is not rushed. The soul's timing does not adhere to the way we are taught in Western cultures to move through the death and dying process. When we do not allow time for our inner being to catch up to what is happening, we get stuck, and that becomes a trauma that is carried into the future.

As a death doula, your work makes room for slowing things down. You make room for the shock of death, and by supporting it, you help to prevent it from turning into a traumatic event. Your work provides the structure for the person in their dying time and those that surround them so their inner being can catch up and come to terms with what is taking place in front of them.

ACKNOWLEDGE THE INEXPLICABLE

Not only are the changes in the way time moves at the deathbed noticeable, but so are other changes in the environment surrounding the dying person that require a certain flexibility in perception and willingness to be open to that which is unknown to us. As you begin your work as a death doula, you will start to develop ways to see what is hidden from those who do not have the ears or eyes to see what is present in the dying space. Some may attribute deathbed-related phenomena as coincidences or tricks your brain is playing to make sense of an intense situation. It is up to you to use your senses and decide what you are witnessing. Speaking from my own personal experience, no one needs to validate the phenomena you experience when someone dies.

Death-related phenomena can include changes in light levels of the room, as though a loving light fills the space. The air temperature of the space can change. My experience has always been of the room growing colder in spots temporarily. The air in the room can become heavy and can take longer to clear. People speak of having seen vapors leave the body of the deceased. Pets can begin to act out of character, assuming that they are more in tune with the subtle changes of their environments than we humans are. I have even read stories of clocks stopping, although I have never had that happen to me. Birds or butterflies can even appear at the windows after the time of death.

You may have had strange occurrences happen when you lost someone dear to you and not allowed yourself permission to see it as related to the person's passing. Maybe someone in your life dismissed the experience, but you still hold on to the idea that there was meaning in the experience. Maybe, in fact, it was a coincidence that something abnormal happened when someone you loved passed away. Does it really matter if it was real or not if it brings you comfort or creates a cherished memory? Like I stated before, you do not need to validate the phenomena that take place at a person's dying time.

Sometimes the strange event that takes place is the fact that you were not able to be at the person's bedside. It is as though something was preventing you from being there or that the dying person deliberately waited until you left the room to die. The day that my mother began to die, as I worked on traveling from my home in Colorado to her in

Indiana, it seemed like the world was conspiring against me getting to the hospital on time. Booking my airline ticket was problematic; there was more traffic than usual on the way to the airport; the gate agent could not find my plane ticket in the system; security was backed up; I arrived at the gate just in time to board the plane and take the window seat in the very last aisle of the plane. There were also things that worked in my favor to get me to my mom in time too. Once I laid my head on the counter and told the gate agent why I was traveling, she buckled down and found my ticket. She shoved the ticket in my hand, hugged me, and firmly pushed me on my way. Then at airport security, the long line was halved when a friend waved me up further and asked why I was traveling. Any person who had complained that I jumped the line immediately changed their tune when I said, "I am going home because my mom is dying today." So it seemed as though I would make it to see my mom in person before she died, that I could be with her and my family while she passed away. I felt as though the world was trying to prevent me from getting there, while the people in it were working to make sure I made it in time.

It would not be so, though. With an hour left on my flight, my big sister told my mom that she only had to wait one more hour and that I would be home. My sister probably thought as I did that my mom would want to be in both of her daughter's physical presence while dying. Nope. As soon as my sister uttered those words to my mom, her vitals started dropping, and in less than the time it was going to take me to get to the hospital, my mom was gone. Both my sister and I believe that our mother made a choice. She had always tried to shield me from harm when I was a kid; why would she act any differently now that she was dying? It was a choice that she made.

There are times when the dying person makes a choice as

to whom they want in the space when they pass away. A loving husband married for fifty-plus years will wait until his wife decides to take the nurse's guidance and go home to shower and nap. As soon as she is far enough away from the nursing home that she cannot make a quick return if notified, the husband dies. A grandmother lying in bed with her two grown granddaughters sitting in the room begins to release from her body and begins to tell who or whatever spirit came for her to "go, get out of here" after not speaking for days. She then dies the next morning before her daughter arrives and only her son is present as though she was protecting her youngest child and granddaughters from seeing her die. A normally private person in life is not able to relax enough to slip from their body on their deathbed until the room is less crowded with people. Now, can these circumstances be categorized as coincidence? Maybe. Possibly. Sure, why not? But if we open our minds to the idea that we do not know everything about death and allow for mystery and miracles to enter, then these events can be seen as purposeful and chosen.

By developing your senses, opening your mind to the range of possibilities, and finding meaning in things hidden from those who have not the ability to receive, you will start to see the magic in the dying experience. By no means does the magic take away the pain, sadness, boredom, or negative emotions that come along with being with someone who is dying; instead, the magic runs parallel to them.

THEORIES ABOUT DEATH AND DYING

When it comes to preparing for death and dealing with the grieving process, there are many theories that broaden our understanding of an individual's impression of what is taking place.

Identifying how a person has formed attachments to individuals and objects in their lives can help the death doula support them as they surrender connections to their physical life. Knowing the language used and the theories that explore the human experience of the dying and grieving process are key to implementing the skills of doula. Put simply, you will need to have an idea of why people are acting the way they are, where any resistance is, and what supports can be put in place to walk with your clients through their dying process. Just like with medical terminology relating to death, these concepts do not have to be memorized word for word and you do not have to memorize the names. There is no written test on this material. What does need to happen is an integration of the material presented through reflection and lived experience. Ideas from human sciences such as psychology, sociology, divinity, and theology are relevant to a death doula's work, but having advanced training in the areas is not required. The death doula is not there to diagnose or fix anything in the dying journey. The art of being a death doula is about being with a person at their most vulnerable time and providing holistic support for their journey.

MASLOW'S HIERARCHY OF NEEDS

Abraham Maslow's psychology theory published in 1943 in the paper "A Theory of Human Motivation" (http://psychclassics.yorku.ca/Maslow/motivation.htm) is made up of an eight-level triangle with the most fundamental physical needs shown at the bottom and the personal fulfillment needs of self-actualization and transcendence at the top. The pyramid is arranged in a hierarchy with needs lower down needing to be satisfied before people can begin to attend to needs higher up on the pyramid. The theory illustrates the needs starting with the bottom of the pyramid to the top:

- Biological and physiological needs or basic life needs: air, food, water, warmth, sleep

- Safety needs: protection, security, order, laws, limits, stability

- Belongingness and love needs: family, affection, relationships, work, group

- Esteem needs: achievement, status, responsibility, reputation

- Cognitive needs: knowledge, meaning, self-awareness

- Aesthetic needs: beauty, balance, form

- Self-actualization: personal growth, fulfillment, transcendence

Maslow's hierarchy of needs pyramid is a popular theory to approach human behavior. It can be used as a good starting point for understanding why people behave as they do, but it is not a perfect theory. Because of its popularity in explaining human behaviors, a death doula should have an understanding of it and what it means for their work. How this idea applies to your work as a doula is that we can recognize how dying people and their surrounding circles may struggle with different issues depending on where they fall on the pyramid.

Looking at the people you work with through this lens may be informative, but the situation and the people involved are not always that simple. Take, for instance, going to a homeless campsite to help a man who has lived on the streets for the majority of his adult life die peacefully. You might first think that this man would be categorized on the lowest level of the pyramid because he is lacking security and some basic physical needs like a home, that he will not need to talk about the other needs on the hierarchy pyramid. While that may be true, 100 percent completion of each level is not necessary to attain merits of a higher level. A dying person, no matter their living condition or what level they may be at on a psychological measure of fulfillment or value, deserves the dignity of a supported death. Working with dying people encompasses all that you can learn in multiple specialties full of technical terms while also being idea-shattering.

Even more helpful to death doulas is how Maslow's pyramid can be applied to the care of the dying person. You'll notice needs change as a person begins to transition away from life. Restructuring the pyramid to account for the needs of the dying looks like this starting with the bottom of the pyramid moving to the top:

- The most basic need to meet in a dying person's experience is controlling and providing comfort for symptoms that make the dying process more difficult, in other words: comfort care. The goal of comfort care is not to extend a person's life but to ease difficult symptoms.

- Next, assure them of their physical safety by alleviating the dying's fears of abandonment and providing a space for them to transition. In the homeless man's case, this was not a hospital or suburban home but a tent where he had been living.

- The third pyramid layer allows for acceptance, love, and affection in the face of death. For many people, their dying time is a time when they are closeted away because of others' discomfort and unwillingness to acknowledge that death is near. It can be a time full of fear leading to the inability to look dying people in the face, which causes the dying person to not feel accepted and forgotten. It is important to remember that dying is still living.

- The fourth layer of the adapted pyramid includes respect, esteem, and appreciation of the person. This layer is where the stories and gratitude live.

- At the top of the pyramid are transcendence and self-actualization. This can be described as the actual death of a person or the surrender and/ or acceptance of death.

Much of the Western world is centered around these ideas of individualism and self-actualization. In fact, Maslow most likely developed his theory after spending time with the Sikiska or Blackfoot First Nation in Canada years before he published his paper. There are many differences between the two. One major difference between Maslow's theory and the Blackfoot Nation's perspective is Maslow's omission of any talk of community actualization. Community is often left out of the Western culture's ideas because of the intense focus on the individual. But no one is an island unto themselves. Even if we do not interact with people in our community, we are still a part of that community. We are all connected regardless of how individually focused our thoughts and ideas are.

Understanding how one person's death affects a community is a major part of what the death doula does. Whether "community" is used to describe a family, a friend group, or people who live in the same area as the dying person, the death doula recognizes and addresses that one single death affects many. While it is important to understand theories such as Maslow's Hierarchy of Needs that are often used when it comes to the human experience, as death doulas, we need to dig deeper into other cultural worldviews to support what is being witnessed in our work. Western worldviews often impose limitations on the dying journey and the grieving process. It is our job as death doulas to allow space for the true experience and expression instead of strictly adhering to ideas and theories about life and death.

KUBLER-ROSS STAGES OF DEATH AND DYING

Dr. Elizabeth Kubler-Ross's five stages of grieving – denial, anger, bargaining, depression, and acceptance – create a framework for how we learn to come to terms with being told a person is going to die and how people live without the ones they have lost. Kubler-Ross's work was created as an outline to help understand how a dying person emotionally moves through their dying process.

Examples for how the emotions can show up in the dying space include:

- Grief felt in many forms on all ends of the dying journey – grief felt by the one who is dying as they come to terms with their mortality and grief felt by those who remain.

- When a person is in a state of shock, they feel numb, closed off, empty, and express dread. Denial often sets in when a person feels shock and disbelief possibly as a way to express self-preservation that may feel mildly comforting.

- Deep pain and guilt are often experienced, which can cause people to attempt to get closer to those in their lives or do the opposite and to pull away.

- Feelings of anger may surface as people question why they are dying.

- Bargaining is the "if" and "should have" stage where guilt and vulnerability come out. It is when people may express how they wished they would have done things differently.

- Depression may be expressed as great sadness, hopelessness, frustration, and loneliness.

- Acceptance and hope are usually when the dying person grows to accept that they are indeed going to die and strive to connect to something bigger than themselves before their death comes.

The stages are used to recognize and identify what people may be feeling. They do not create a linear timeline for emotions during the dying process. Not everyone goes through all of them or in a prescribed order. Grief is unique. Emotional processing is unique. By understanding the stages in the theory, the death doula can begin to identify what a person may need from them at a certain point in time. Death doulas can model how it is to be with grief and distressing emotions by not rushing to fix the situation, by not forcing people to move through their emotions faster than they are ready to, and by being available for when someone is ready to share about their experience or just be present with them.

STACKING GRIEF

> *"Grief expressed out loud, whether in or out of character, un-choreographed and honest, for someone we have lost, or a country or home we have lost, is in itself the greatest praise we could ever give them. Grief is praise because it is the natural way love honors what it misses."*
>
> — MARTIN PRECHTEL

Grief is commonly thought of as something that people do after someone has died. Grief actually shows up for every little loss that occurs along the dying process. When sitting with a circle of people filled with family or friends that is supporting a dying person's transition, it is easy to see that grieving is not something that starts after a person has ceased to live.

Francis Weller, author and psychotherapist, talks about grief being a threshold emotion. Once we cross the threshold and walk into the room of grief, we begin to allow ourselves to actively mourn. The act has a way of opening up our lived experience to a wider range of sensations and emotions. It is an emotional process of healing. I have often heard people say, "What you can feel, you can heal." Your work as a death doula will allow the people in the dying space to begin to feel their emotions instead of rushing through them or brushing them off. This is one way our work becomes an instrument of healing.

Grieving is an active process. It is made up of feelings. We all have preferences for how we express our emotions, including grief. Maybe the way emotion is expressed by a person is not chosen but learned instead.

DIFFERENT TYPES OF GRIEF

Another consideration for assisting those in the dying process and those in the circle that surround them is the type of grief they are experiencing. Are they able to actively grieve? Is their grief suspended due to some separation? Are they being passive or inhibiting their grief and not allowing it to be expressed? Although not every dying person needs to pick apart the emotions they feel during their dying time, it will be helpful for you, as their death doula, to notice what they are going through and inquire about it. Remember, it is not your job to fix the situation. You cannot fix the fact that this person in front of you is going to die. You can only make room for all the complicated, beautiful, and painful feelings that come up. That is a gift you can give to a dying person and their circles of people.

Let us dig a little deeper into the different types of grief to give you another perspective on why people behave how they do in the dying space. How their actions are affected by how they are able to grieve or not grieve during the dying process. Having knowledge and awareness of the different types of grief can help support yourself because you will not be free from feeling intense emotions while serving dying people. Plus, understanding different types of grief will help you if your work involves supporting people after a death has occurred through creating rituals or providing grief support.

Active grief is defined most simply as openly admitting that something has been lost, that life has changed. It can be characterized by crying. This allows our bodies to release hormones related to regulating stress and anxiety. This way of mourning permits the person to begin to let go of the one they have lost and begin to establish a new relationship with their deceased loved one. Oh yes, relationships do not have to end just because one person is no longer on the earthly plane of existence.

Acute grief pertains to the period immediately following the death of a loved one that can be characterized by a person's loss of emotional and physical regulation. An increased intensity and frequency of anger, sadness, anxiety, feeling numb, and difficulty concentrating also characterize this type of grief. Sleep schedules can be disrupted. The desire to eat can also diminish. This type of grief can show up as what I call a "grief collapse" or the body of the griever physically collapsing upon hearing upsetting news. It can also show up as anger at the world and the people in it for continuing on after upsetting news is received.

Complicated grief, complicated grief disorder, or prolonged grief disorder can be categorized as someone experiencing grief of a greater intensity that does not improve over time and is severe enough to affect a person's ability to return to normal activities. Complicated grief disorder even appears in the Diagnostic and Statistical Manual - 5 (DSM-5) used by psychiatrists and clinicians. This type of grief may need support from a therapist and possibly medication, but it most definitely requires patience and nonjudgement from those around the grieving person. This type of grief can also be labeled as unresolved grief. This type of grief can present more easily in people with low self-esteem and a complicated relationship with self.

Inhibited or absent grief is the suppression or denial of overt expressions of grief. The lack of expression of intense emotions does not imply that the person does not experience feelings associated with grief. The person, however, willingly or unwillingly is choosing to not give the feelings much time. It also shows up as not outwardly sharing emotions with others. Inhibiting one's grief can be due to a person not being able to face their loved one's death. Actively ignoring one's grief can have physical and emotional consequences later in life. I find that when people do not allow themselves to experience grief, even in its smallest expression, that it will act like water moving down a river. Eventually, the water will find a way whether it be through a rock or over a dam; it will flow out and maybe at a time that is not convenient.

Suspended grief is exactly as it sounds. A person is not fully able to experience their grief because closure or connection has not been had. Their grief hangs in a limbo state of feeling like they do not have all the pieces needed to fully grieve. This is commonly experienced when someone is not able to be physically present with their dear person at their dying time. This can also happen when funerals or ceremonies are not able to take place. Suspended grief can feel confusing because of lack of information in the case of traumatic deaths or death by suicide; it can also feel like a person is carrying an unnamed hole in their heart that physical connection or ceremony could fill.

Disenfranchised grief is grief that goes unwitnessed. It is hidden maybe because the person experiencing it feels guilty for having it or maybe they worry that what they are mourning is not a significant event like the death of a pet. Disenfranchised grief is anything that is not validated by social norms. It shows up in loss for those in unrecognized relationships such as nontraditional romantic partnerships or intense love felt for a nonromantic partner. It can show up in unacknowledged personal identifications such as gender identification. No being able to mourn the loss of pets or other events considered less significant by some falls into the realm of disenfranchised grief. This type of grief also holds those who are socially excluded from showing grief or who are considered incapable of grieving.

Grief is something that we actively do, even by avoiding it; it is also something that we carry. I believe that when someone dear to us dies or even someone with whom we have a complicated relationship passes away, that grief does not leave us. Its expression may change over time, but still, it remains. How it affects us oscillates daily.

Over the course of a lifetime, a person stacks their experienced grief. Their past reactions to losses and how they held the experience can impact how they process current difficulties. For me, my stacked grief and lived experiences showed up one night at the hospital when my team was caring for an elderly woman. Seeing how thin, frail, and ill the lady was took me right back to my grandmother's dying time. It returned my grief and took my breath away. It felt like a punch to the gut. The two women looked similar in their thinness and how they positioned their bodies in much the same fashion. What came up for me took me by surprise as my grandmother had passed away many years before, and I was not unhappy with my mourning process for her. I noticed that what I was feeling was not related to my grandmother's death but the care before her death. Our patient's appearance and health condition elicited a response in me that caused me to create a story in my mind that was similar to someone I loved. Was the story true? It was for my grandmother, but I do not have any idea if it was for our elderly patient. My biggest takeaway from this quick return of grief was that there were parts of losing my grandmother that I still needed to work on and that I carried anger over her care. Did recognizing this fix the way I was feeling? Absolutely not, but it made me aware of how events that I thought I was done with could affect my current situation.

Understanding that grief may be stacked and carried over a lifetime is important to the work of the death doula because the people we serve will bring a lifetime of experiences and emotions to the dying space. Emotions that show up in the dying space may be deeply connected to something in the past. While we may not be able to resolve what occurred, we can provide a safe space for people to allow themselves to own that the event has had an effect on their life and then guide them as they work to let it go during the dying process.

THE LANGUAGE OF THE SOUL

Much distress that comes at a person's dying time is due to the inner turmoil that they feel. Death brings so much which is unknown and asks a person to leave so much behind. How can we possibly walk with people as they begin to release and let go of their lives? The work of doing this begins with acknowledging the many complex layers that people experience death in. Dying is not just a religious or physical event. It involves all of our human existence, our cognitive life, our emotional life, our physical bodies, and our relationship to spirit.

The language of the soul removes the confusion that we have over our existence being singularly connected to our physical body. When we allow room for people to journey through their dying time in a way that acknowledges more layers, we build a container that not only helps them to not feel alone but to feel connected and maybe even healed. The potential to heal comes from bringing together all the layers of the dying experience.

PAIN AND RELAXING INTO DEATH

Death, like giving birth, requires labor. The effort of dying can be impeded by physical, emotional, and spiritual distress. If there is unfinished business in life, the labor of death can take longer. If there is a great amount of physical pain, then the dying person will be unable to relax into the experience and may fight their dying time. Fear and other emotions can also slow things down. The work of the death doula can provide support in the laboring process. In future chapters, you will begin to learn tools to help the people you support ease into the dying process.

For those surrounding the dying person, the moment of death can be intensely spiritual, profound, and/ or uncomfortable. Death can seem anticlimactic after all the stress and time spent waiting for it to occur. The body can seem like an empty envelope after someone passes away. Those in the dying space can be left to feel numb, relief, anger, confusion... There is no right or wrong way to feel after a death. All emotions are valid. Your work as a doula will model this idea by increasing your ability to be present with a wide range of emotions of others and your own.

While it is not the goal of the death doula to fix what is being experienced in the dying space, it is a goal to allow for conscious awareness of the experience, to be authentic, honest, and gentle with all in the dying circle. By being a model for conscious awareness and true emotional expression, you will become a tool of healing and sacredness for those present in the dying space.

In order to begin working with what is present in the dying space, the death doula must first develop their ability to acutely notice/ observe what is going on in their environment and within the people present there. The exercises at the end of this chapter will help you begin to develop your noticing skills by observing your surroundings and by working with stories that people tell. Practicing these exercises will help you begin to see subtle connections in the world around you.

Once you further develop your noticing skills, you may start observing that humans are all connected and that behaviors, emotions, and energy levels are just as catching as yawning is. You may see what French chemist Antione-Laurent Lavoisier said, "Nothing's created. Nothing's lost. Everything changes to another form."

Western science and culture are beginning to accept the idea that everything is connected and that nothing truly goes away. Proof of unseen connections between living things is being identified in work with humans and their environment and also by scientists who are identifying the way trees communicate with each other. This interconnected worldview of living has been long held by many much older cultures and ways of medicine. As a death doula, you can begin to weave the knowledge of Western medical practices and ways of being with more comprehensive worldviews that accept that one life is a small part of something bigger.

In the next chapter, you will take this idea and add it to the skills needed to cocreate a deathbed ecosystem that supports the dying person and all people present in the dying space.

DEATH DOULA STARTER PACK

How do you express grief exercise?

1. How do you express grief? It might be easier to go through this by thinking about how and when you cry.

Do you cry openly in front of others when you are hurt or sad? How about when you are injured or sick? Or are you like me and want to cry in private?

I admit it: I am a bathroom crier. It does not mean that I do not acknowledge my feelings in the moment. I just choose to release those feelings in private.

Acknowledging and releasing emotions are two separate actions. This can happen in a split second and feel like there is no control over it, and it can also be a deliberate choice in the moment. I have not always had the choice to wait privately to have an emotional release – the trigger for the emotional reaction may have been too intense – but I have noticed it is what I prefer. Neither crying in public or crying in private is right or wrong. It is about what works for the individual. Many times, when the crying seems to not work, in fact, it is not because of what the crying person is feeling. It is because the expression makes those around the crying person uncomfortable. Crying, just like grief, is rushed to be comforted because many people cannot withstand the uneasy feeling they get being around someone actively expressing their emotions.

2. Think about a situation where you saw someone expressing an uncomfortable emotion, like a teen releasing disappointment over not getting cast in a role they auditioned for. How quickly do the people surrounding the teenager try to ease or eliminate their pain only to see that the attempt to rush the feelings only makes the teen more

upset? Why are we taught to rush through our feelings, especially those we are taught that are negative?

Let's again reference yourself and take a moment to reflect on how you show grief. How has grief shown up for you when you lost someone dear to you? You may have come to read this book as someone who has yet to be with a dying person. You are lucky enough to not have gone through the death of someone near and dear to you. You may think that you have never felt grief and have no idea how you process all that comes with it. That is when we begin to look for parallel experiences.

Parallel Intensity Experience Exercise

Go back to envisioning a mild to medium intensity level crying episode that you have had. By that, I mean something that elicits a response when you think about it but nothing so intense that it makes you unable to complete the exercise.

- What caused the crying episode?

- What other emotions came up?

- What did you do physically with your body?

- Did it help you to feel better?

This same exercise can be done with various emotions like anger, feeling overwhelmed, happiness, or even feeling tired. It can also be helpful to ask yourself these questions and substitute another person's reactions for your own. Practicing this is not about getting the answers right or wrong. Instead, you are working on strengthening your muscle to be with or acknowledge and understand the emotional journeys of others, whether it be through grief or joy.

What are you feeling in your body right now?

This practice can be completed with two people or on your own. It can be interesting to do this with your partner or with a child.

First, have the person tell a story about an experience they have had. Make sure that the experience is not overly intense. It can be a positive or negative experience but keep it a mild to medium experience to ensure the exercise can be completed.

If you are working with a partner, complete the following:

What I saw was…

What I heard or did not hear was…

What I felt or did not feel was…

What I sensed was…

Is any of that accurate?

What I wonder is…

Allow the first speaker to reflect back their experience of this practice.

Working on your own, begin this practice by recalling a mild to medium experience. Allow yourself to relive it in your mind. Now, ask yourself the same questions. Reflect back on the experience and see if it was accurate and if you noticed anything different about it.

The Field

What is not being said but still being heard? Look around and begin to notice what the space you are in is communicating to you. You can tell a lot by what objects are in a room.

Take time to get an idea about how the space feels. Are there other people in the room? If so, what can you learn by observing them? Really allow yourself to take it all in. Are you able to pick up on others' energy levels by watching them? Or are you able to feel others' energy levels? As you strengthen your noticing skills, you will begin to watch not only for what people are saying with language and their bodies but also for what is being communicated in the environment. Reading the field provides a way to scan the surrounding, take into consideration other people's perspectives and what information they are putting out into the world, and attune yourself to them regardless of time spent together.

So, how do we go about learning how to read the field and become a super noticer?

- Open yourself up to be curious about yourself and others
- Read facial, vocal, and body language
- Notice the absence or presence of feelings
- Read or sense emotional tones
- Watch for mismatched stories and feelings
- Be aware of your own emotions
- Find words to describe how you are observing
- Add visual details as if painting a picture if able to
- Get a feeling for the energy of the space

6

DEFINING THE DEATHBED ECOSYSTEM

"The art of dying well starts with the art of living well."

— L.S. DUGDALE

As mentioned in previous chapters, death does not consist of only one giant loss; instead, the dying journey consists of multiple little losses that lead to the final loss. It can be referred to as the indignities suffered by the dying person. The moments leading up to death are overflowing with changes: diminished body capabilities, withdrawal from communities and activities that have provided purpose, loss of meaning for those whose focus has been on the external life, relocation of house and home, having basic needs met by others. These smaller losses can lead to existential crises for the dying person. This is why people facing death so often suffer from depression and/ or anxiety. Who wouldn't at the thought of their entire world potentially changing only to lead to some unknown experience?

It is here that we can begin to implement the subtle doula

arts and help those we support by building a deathbed ecosystem that takes into account the whole person. The deathbed ecosystem creates a holistic values-based care plan that is made up of physical things that we can touch and the ethereal aspects that honor the essence of the dying person. At its most basic level, the deathbed ecosystem is made up of tangible aspects – the physical environment the person will be in, the people that are present, and how those people will interact in the environment. The more complex side of the deathbed ecosystem identifies and defines the intangibles – the feelings behind the actions that bring comfort in life and how to softly hold how hard the experience while not diminishing it.

The work of creating a deathbed ecosystem starts before many death doulas enter into a supportive relationship with their clients when the medical and financial end of life paperwork is completed. While some of the creation of this paperwork can be completed with a death doula, it is a task that may need the support of a lawyer, financial advisor, and/ or doctor. A link to an overview of the paperwork and other end-of-life terminology can be found at the end of the book.

As a death doula, you will begin the work of creating a deathbed ecosystem by having courageous conversations and by engaging in deep listening. To map out what is in a person's deathbed ecosystem, the death doula needs to be highly skilled in communication. In this chapter, you will learn how to develop advanced conversational practices that will help you identify what is needed to create a guide for the care and keeping of your clients by building trust and safety in your relationship. You will learn how your personal state of being can influence your interactions and how to manage that. You will also learn the importance of speaking to people in their own language and how it moves the relationship forward. Once you have begun to implement the deep conversation skills, you can guide your clients to map out the concrete physical aspects of their deathbed ecosystem while integrating the essence of what they value. It all starts with asking questions.

COURAGEOUS CONVERSATIONS

> *"Thanks to the human heart by which we live,*
> *Thanks to its tenderness, its joys, and fears.*
> *To me, the meanest flower that blows can give*
> *thoughts that do often lie too deep for tears."*
>
> — WILLIAM WORDSWORTH

The first step in creating the deathbed ecosystem is having courageous conversations. As doulas, we cannot map out the ecosystem without first getting to know our clients. The way we get to know them is by simply talking to them.

Most people move through life never truly listening to those around them. It is as though we as a culture are conditioned to have our minds focused on our responses instead of fully hearing what is being conveyed to us. This is a common occurrence when what someone is speaking about is uncomfortable to hear, like when someone talks about life-limiting changes they are going through at end of life. This conversational space is where the intangible side of the deathbed ecosystem first develops. This is where the skills of a death doula shine. In order to have courageous conversations, the death doula should be skilled in all the components that make up effective communication: the energy of communication, listening, and language.

In the early moments of courageous conversations, it is

important to practice the ability to quiet your own mind, your personal fears, and truly listen with your whole being. So, before you go headfirst into an intense conversation with someone, take a moment to ensure that your personal life and your thoughts will not interfere in the exchange. Think of it as quieting your internal chatter. I will discuss ways of doing this more in Chapter 8.

It is also important to check in on how you are communicating energetically before you begin the conversation. All forms of communication carry energy in them. Work to develop a self-awareness of the energy of your exchanges with people.

ENERGY OF COMMUNICATION

> *"We are always communicating energetically expressions to others. We are influencing self, others, and the world positively or negatively all the time."*
>
> — CONSCIOUS DYING INSTITUTE

The energy we put into our communication and the emotions we carry inside of us color the way we interact. As doulas, we must act a grounding force during the turbulent time of the dying process. It is thought that all humans have an energy field that surrounds them. The HeartMath Institute's research shows that the human heart carries energy that can be detected by others. Dr. Rollin McCraty, psychophysiologist and director of research at HeartMath Institute says, "The heart generates the largest electromagnetic field in the body. The electrical field measured in an electrocardiogram (ECG) is about sixty times greater in amplitude than the brain waves recorded in an electroencephalogram (EEG)." This is a source of our subtle yet influential electromagnetic or "energetic" communication system operating just below our conscious level of awareness. Communication takes place even when we are not speaking. Our bodies pick up energy signals from the environment, nature, and those around us. This is why we feel uplifted when we are around positive people or down when we are surrounded by negative people. Energy is felt even when it cannot be explained.

It only takes one person to be the source of good energy or to be the example for fully embracing all of the feelings that come up in the dying space. The death doulas can bring both to the deathbed ecosystem by being an amplifier for the wishes of the person in their dying time.

Dr. Sarah Kerr, whom I've mentioned before, refers to it this way: "When we walk into a room to perform a ritual with a family, we carry that energy. It is not because we know it and we can explain it. It's because we live it. It's wired into our energy."

LISTENING

Now that your inner being is in the right place, you can enter into a courageous conversation with the person you are supporting. The first rule of being part of a courageous conversation, as I already hinted at, is listening. As a death doula, you will work to hear what is said not just with your ears but your whole being, your body, mind, heart, and spirit. You will also work to hear what is not being said. I can tell you from experience that it is not helpful to "machine gun" questions at people even though that could be a quick way to gather information. Very few people like a succession of rapid-fire questions. Instead, give the conversation time and space to develop. Even though your client's time is limited, it is essential to make them feel expansive in the conversation.

Listening can be broken down in multiple ways. It is important to note that listening and asking questions are closely tied to one another. Unless you are open to fully hearing what a person has to say, you cannot form a high level of trust. Lack of trust will cause the person to be less willing to be vulnerable in answering your questions. As a death doula, your ability to listen will quickly become one of your greatest services that you can provide to people in their dying time. Listening is underrated. Many people listen in order to form a great response instead of listening to understand what is being said. Our inability to set aside our next statement prevents us from being fully present with another person. It can make a person feel lonely when what they have to say is rushed over in an attempt to fix whatever is mentioned.

Broken down into its components, listening is made up of pure listening, basic listening, and active listening.

With pure listening, you are listening with your presence to understand. You sit in total awareness of what the other person is saying, but you do not respond. At its most pure level, you are just being with the other person. You are not pushing their train of thought in any direction with your questions. You are allowing their words to flow from them by not giving them the answers or interrupting their thoughts. Occasionally, pure listening takes the form of silence. Even if the person you are supporting is not willing to talk or is past the point in the dying process of speaking, they still have things to communicate. With practice, you will be able to understand what the person is saying with their body language, breathing patterns, and energy. Your ability to notice will increase the more time you spend in quiet whole-body observation.

Basic listening is what most people are accustomed to doing. It is a back-and-forth between people using words or gestures, but it involves more shallow topics, questions, and less deep presence. While this level of listening can be good at times, it is not deep enough to consistently use in your daily work as a death doula. There will be times when you engage in basic listening, and that is okay. I often use this style of listening when I have warm-up conversations with people. Not many people are willing early in the process of setting up a deathbed ecosystem to start directly speaking of death. Serious topics often deserve a conversational warm-up.

Basic listening exchanges are often good when first establishing a relationship with the person you will be serving. They are also good for warming people with whom you have been in a relationship with but now because of the circumstances, the power dynamic has changed, or they are not comfortable with being vulnerable.

Being a death doula is not about being perfect in your skills at all times. It is instead about being spacious in your way of thinking and doing things. What I mean by spacious is that you practice a gentleness in the way you evaluate yourself and with the way you interact with others. Conversations will not always go as you hope; you may not always succeed in providing comfort the way it is needed, and the people you serve are not going to be able to get out of dying. So, remember to give grace where it is needed, starting with yourself.

What you will engage in most of the time with the people you support will be deep, active listening. This type of listening will not occur if a relationship of trust and safety has not been established prior to diving deep with questions. While many of the people you work with will have a limited amount of time for you to work with them, any other skills you have to offer, any other forms of comfort that you can provide are secondary to establishing trust and safety. Dying people are vulnerable on many levels. It is paramount for death doulas to quickly see the places where people are feeling exposed and fragile, let them know that you are a safe person to be with, and gently support them at their level.

In the dying process, there are many ideas about different stages, emotions, or experiences that people will journey through. While that sounds nice on paper, in life, it does not always happen. You may find yourself serving a person who has no want of what you have to offer, especially if you are in a volunteer situation or with a family member who has not agreed to receive what you can provide. Do not be pushy with your offerings in these situations, but find a way to give. Meet them where they are. If they do not want to talk about their death, fine, do that, but still be with them. Talk to them about things that they do want to talk about. Deep conversations are not better for every person, but every person deserves someone who will listen to whatever they have to say deeply.

Active listening is important when interacting with the dying because we do not want them to feel alone in their experience. They are already alone in the fact that they will soon leave their body, but they do not have to feel lonely by not being heard. Allow the people in the dying space to speak their truth. Do not assume what they are feeling. This applies to the person who is dying and also to those surrounding them.

LANGUAGE

When you begin to engage in deep active listening, you will incorporate pure listening with your whole being and add to it reflecting what you have heard to check for accuracy and understanding. This is a time to speak the language of the person you are with. Use the same phrases that they use; sprinkle in some of the exact words they have used to describe what they are expressing. Try to subtly mirror their body language, hand gestures, and the rhythm of their speech.

Ask open-ended questions. Limit questions that can be answered with a simple yes or no. Try to refrain from giving advice or directing the person's response right away. People work with death doulas to receive advice and guidance on how to traverse their dying time, but it is difficult to serve our people if we do not fully hear what someone is saying.

One way to ensure that you as the death doula have truly heard what people are saying is to ask clarifying questions. I like the practice of asking someone to explain what they are experiencing from their point of view. Follow up their explanation by stating in your own words what you heard them say and then ask if it is correct. Keep doing this until the person you are speaking with feels understood. Another good question to ask for greater understanding is simply why. "Why do you feel that way?" Why do you think that?"

Don't make the mistake that I have made and rapid-fire questions at people while not allowing them time to respond. And remember, the people that you are talking to may have things they want to share with you that you did not ask about. It is easy to give them permission to share those things by simply asking, "Is there anything else?"

I like to open sessions with a few warm-up questions. If it is my first time working with someone, the questions are more of a get-to-know-you flavor. If we have worked together before, I give them some time to get me caught up on how life is going for them. I allow them time to tell stories about the people in their lives. It takes practice to integrate this type of opener into your sessions without the warm-up questions and sharing taking over the whole session. Sometimes, all the person you are serving needs is to chat with someone who fully sees them as they are while they are dying.

SESSION-OPENING QUESTIONS

- How has your day been today?
- How can I serve you today?
- How did you feel after our last session together?
- Is there anything that you would like to do differently today?
- Is there anything causing you pain or anxiety?

DEFINING THEIR WORDS

Another important part of having courageous conversations is getting the meaning behind a person's words. Take the word "cheap," for example. When I, a person firmly in the middle class, buy something and say that it was cheap, it is probably different than when Oprah buys something and says it is cheap.

With spoken language, we use words that reflect much of our lived experiences. Our personal histories, our unique ways of interpreting our feelings and experiences, our family of origin, and our cultural background are factors that influence our word selection.

Words have definite meanings. They often have multiple definitions, but we cannot assume to know how a person using the word is intending the word choice to be understood. Now, this is not meant to be a dissection of the language. The intention here is for the death doula to understand that they need to get clarification on certain words their clients use.

The best way to explain is by talking about quality of life. Quality of life means different things to different people. You will not accurately know what a person's definition is until you ask questions to focus their answer. It is easy to base another's definition on your own idea of what something means to you. For one person, quality can mean as long as they can be with their family; even if they are on a ventilator, they want to live. For another, not being able to walk is too far from their idea of quality life.

You may choose the words you speak, but you do so based on what you learned in school, at home, on the internet, or in your social interactions. The words we choose to say can have multiple definitions, and they can mean different things to different people. The differences in meanings that people apply to words make it especially important for you as the death doula to ask clarifying questions about descriptors that are used by people to explain their feelings or experiences. For example, a woman sitting with a parent on hospice is told by her mother's nurse after checking her vital signs that her mom is doing "great." The woman instantly questions "great" in her mind. How can her mom be doing "great" when she is dying? What the nurse meant and what she said were two different things. The nurse knew that the "great" meant that the mother's vital signs were not fluctuating, that they were consistent with where the patient was at in the dying process. The daughter had no idea that was how the nurse meant her statement. Her only thought upon hearing "great" was that her mother's condition was improving and that she might not in fact be dying.

The lesson here is to choose your words to accurately describe what is happening in a way that those in the deathbed ecosystem understand. It does not serve the dying person or the people supporting them to use unclear or difficult to interpret language. It is also relevant to consider that some words and terms work for certain people but not for others. Healthcare professionals operate in a world full of medical jargon; religious leaders' words are made richer by quoting scripture or religious texts; and people who have done a lot of work in self-development use words like "synchronized" and "integrate" that may confuse others. The ability to meet people where they are and use language that they are familiar with is a skill for the death doula to practice. The words used to explain and comfort an elderly farmer in Winterset, Iowa who is losing his wife may not be the same as the ones used by a middle-aged woman from Boulder, Colorado who reads books on metaphysics extensively. Put more plainly, I do not use the same words when I talk to my spiritual new age friend as I do with my dad. This is referred to as code-switching, which means the practice of shifting the languages you use or the way you express yourself in your conversations depending on who you are speaking to. An example of this was when I compared how what we would say to a rural farmer might be different from a woman interested in metaphysics.

SELECTING YOUR WORDS

Not only do I strive to meet someone where they are at by speaking in terms that are familiar to them, but I also choose my language to reflect the positive influence I am trying to have on the dying experience. One example of this is by changing phrases such as "I have to" to "I get to" do a certain task with an individual. By being thoughtful with our language choices, death doulas provide another layer of authentic care for those they serve while modeling what can occur in the dying space. How we speak about death affects everyone in the deathbed ecosystem and their ability to fully experience death.

By allowing people to explain what is behind their descriptions, you better understand and identify the values they want to uphold in their dying time.

All behavior is communication. The way we move our bodies tells people about us, the tone in our voice conveys emotions, our facial expressions can show hidden feelings, and spoken language can do all of these things but with words.

Death positivity is a phrase that is commonly used in the death trades these days. In my experience, few people are comfortable with this language because few people view death as a positive experience. Talking about death or dealing with death can be overwhelming and uncomfortable for many people. As death doulas, we can embody the death-positive movement while using language that makes more people comfortable.

Our language extends beyond the spoken word. We communicate with our body language and our tone of voice too. Having a soft, calm voice can provide safety in a conversation for those you are speaking with as can mirroring another's body language, speech, facial expression, and more. Mirroring is a mimicking behavior that shows empathy and develops trust. It is often automatic, but with practice, you can consciously use it as a way to put others at ease. When entering into a conversation with someone that you are unfamiliar with, often the people present in the deathbed ecosystem are experiencing a wide range of emotions that can make connecting difficult with a new person. An example of mirroring body movement is crossing your legs after a person next to you does or yawning after someone else yawns.

As a death doula, identifying the intention behind the conversation is another way to people at ease. This can be done by being transparent in your reasons for taking certain actions and explaining the "why" behind them to those present. Identifying intentions also includes mentally evaluating your own actions to ensure that there is not an underlying motivation that does not match what the client desires. Being transparent can involve having gentle conversations with those present in order to clarify their reasons/responses to events. By being transparent and consciously connecting to why you are doing this work before entering the deathbed space, you can open your heart to connect with the hearts of those present. This will begin to develop the level of trust and security needed to build the deathbed ecosystem.

DEFINING QUALITY

One of the first courageous conversations that needs to take place with the people you serve will be to identify what "quality" in "quality of life" means for them. Oftentimes, people will say things like, "When I can no longer feed myself... When I can no longer walk or need help going to the bathroom... then it is done for me." It is important to remember those limitations are some people's starting points in quality of life. Establish what your client's baseline for physical living is – their mobility capabilities, their current disease processes, their hearing, speaking, and vision abilities, any neurological differences, and many more. This is not based on how they were in their body ten years ago – although you can find valuable nuggets of information there –but it is based on how they are physically at the point of diagnosis or when they enter into a supportive relationship with you. Although this part of the conversation is similar in nature to how a medical provider gathers a patient's medical history, it does not have to have the same feeling or proceed the same way. There are things as a death doula that you will not need to know like how many surgeries a person has had, a complete medication list or vitamin list, how many sexual partners a person has had, things that doctors ask for. What will be good to know is what brought them comfort after they had medical procedures in the past? How have they handled being ill? What is soothing to them?

In these conversations, I like to dive into what has brought a person comfort in the past when they experienced illness or for women, when they gave birth. I look for clues. Does the person like touch? What kind of touch? Are there certain smells they enjoy? What kind of noises irritate them or make them happy?

My experience in the operating room taught me that males ranging in ages from teenagers to thirties respond positively and calm down after waking up distressed from surgery when I stroke the corner of their forehead and talk softly to them. The same motion has not elicited the same response from females in the same age group. Also, when working with people with neurodiversity, I have noticed that these topics are especially important. Even when the dying person is no longer able to communicate, it is good to still treat them and the ecosystem that you have co-created with them as though they are still active in it. A human does not have to be sitting up and talking in order to be influenced by their environment.

It will be your job as death doula to learn what kind of physical exchanges the person you are supporting finds comforting, what is off-limits, and marry that with what you are able to provide. You do not have to give the people you help physical touch in order to serve them well, especially if it is not something that you are comfortable with. Remember that you are working to learn what practices work for you and your clients.

One area on another's body that many people are more comfortable with touching are the hands. It can be of great comfort and connection to hold someone's hand while having these courageous conversations after you have established trust.

What else defines quality for a person? The answer can depend on the day, as the dying process is not always linear. It does not always move in one direction, marching toward death. People can improve after a few days of doing poorly, and they can experience rapid changes that limit their comfort and ability to interact with others. The circle of family and friends around a dying person can greatly impact the person's level of comfort and ease in their dying time. Checking in with those surrounding the dying person will allow you to see what is needed in the space by everyone.

ASSESSING THE DAY

In order to gain an idea of what a person's baseline is, it is good to have some questions that you can ask in your early work with a dying person and then small check-ins that you can make later on.

- Describe what a good day is for you.

- What are some things that you like to do on a good day?

- Describe what a bad day is like for you.

- What are some things that are hard for to do you on a bad day?

- Finish this statement: "I want to keep going as long as I can..."

Other areas of comfort that may come up in conversation are access to nature, fresh air, certain light levels, particular smells, or lack of smells, and music. Once, a person I was working with in the early stages of planning mentioned that she wanted to be in the Pacific Northwest during her dying time. She lived in Colorado and had no plans to move, so we shifted the conversation to identifying what it was about the Pacific Northwest that she wanted access to. Through our conversation, we were able to see that it was the trees and air movement that she wanted. In our time together, we also discussed who would be supporting her in her dying time. Her words allowed me to see that she was more comfortable with hiring people to provide for her physical care than relying on her family. She wanted her people to be present with her but not weighed down having to provide for all of her needs. This provided the information that we needed to set up the proper transactional relationships that would meet her physical needs that made room for her family's help if they felt called to assist with her physical needs but did not depend solely on them. Recognizing this allowed us to set up a deathbed ecosystem that was in line with her values and her wishes. She was able to relax and do what she needed to. Dying is hard work. Sitting with the dying is hard too. It is the death doula's job to not take away that fact, but it is our job to hold how hard it is softly and allow for the full range of emotions, connection, and beauty that can occur during the dying process.

DECIDING WHERE

Death is not picky. It will take place wherever. It does not have any space requirements or need any special interior design elements. As a death doula, you will work to identify the ideal place for a person's end of life to unfold and see if this is logistically possible. We can work to provide an environment that meets the physical needs of the dying person while bringing in the essence of their life and what provides them with a measure of whole person comfort. The deathbed ecosystem that you co-create with your client should set them at ease.

With the client I mentioned before who wanted to die in the Pacific Northwest but lived in Colorado, I began to open the courageous conversation to not only the essence of where she wanted to die but bring in what location. Many people state that they want to die at home, but do they know exactly what that involves? Most people do not.

For many, the choice between dying in a facility or at home is not one that they actively make. Without prior talks about this topic, people often end up wherever their dying situation takes them. What that means, where they die is not thoughtfully selected with their input. By saying one wants to die at home, it needs to be taken into consideration if that is physically possible. Does the home provide space for the necessary equipment to support the dying person? Will the layout of the home create challenges while caring for the dying person? Who will meet the needs of the dying person at home? Are the other people that live in the home able and willing to support the dying person in some manner?

Home may not always be the best place to be for them. Medical conditions, limited support, finances, or many other reasons can put someone on the path to spend their last days in a nursing care facility, free-standing hospice facilities, or other medical center. People can also end up moving in with family members, friends, or another group setting to support them in their dying time. None of these locations is better than the other in general. The ideal location for a person to spend their dying days depends on the individual and their circumstances. What is helpful for the person in their dying process is to be able to have a person to talk through their circumstances and identify what their best option is. I have supported people who died at home, used hospice, people who have died in a nursing care facility, people who have died in the hospital, and people who moved in with a friend that could act as their primary caregiver.

In my work, I do advocate for people to use hospice as much as possible. You may decide on something different, but in my opinion, the people who work in hospice are some of the best equipped to deal with the dying process. They live and breathe supporting dying people every day in their work just as death doulas do. And yes, a person can be receiving hospice care and still need a death doula. Why limit the amount of support a person receives?

Another factor in where a person dies and what support services they receive is how near death is. Hospice requires a person to be within six months of death. People can enter hospice care, improve, and graduate out of hospice. A person's dying time most likely will not adhere to a strict timeline.

What medical insurance a person has can also affect where they will spend their dying days. It may be possible that their insurance will cover the costs of dying in a facility better than it will pay for in-home care for those who die at home.

When it comes to working with your client to identify where they will spend their last days, it is important to have them look into what their insurance will cover and what requirements need to be met in order to qualify for that care and talk to the people that they live with and ensure that their family is able and willing to have them die at home.

The essence of home can be brought to any space regardless of where a person chooses to die. If a person chooses not to or is unable to spend their dying days at home, it does not mean that what makes their house a home is unavailable to them. By bringing in elements of what someone attaches to their home to any space, the death doula can recreate a home-like deathbed ecosystem. Often this can be done by bringing photos to place around the room and special mementos to decorate the space. Blankets, pillows, or lamps from home can be brought in, as can books or religious texts the person would like to have nearby. What object is not as important as how it makes the dying person feel.

BUILD A CIRCLE OF COMMUNITY SUPPORT

Another area to address in providing support for a dying person is to identify who will be around them in their dying time. As a teenager, I was permitted to spend a good deal of time with my aunt while she was in the hospital being treated for leukemia. I was even allowed to continue seeing her when it was obvious that she was not going to live through her latest treatment. There did come a point in time when my father decided that I was no longer permitted to see her. Whether I agreed with him or not at the time, I respected his choice. Our family had decided that they did not want the younger people to remember my aunt how she was when she was at her worst physically.

Building a circle of community and family support around a dying person involves these kinds of decisions. Who is the dying comfortable being seen by in their weakest moments? My opinion is that the dying should be shared openly, but my opinions are just that, my opinions. What is most important is what the dying person wants: who they want around them and who the people closest to the dying want around them.

A person's dying time can provide an opportunity for healing relationships or at least providing some kind of closure to interpersonal dynamics. That does not always mean that the people surrounding the dying are in a good place in their relationship with the dying person. That is okay. Perfection is not the goal. Allowing for what is is the goal.

So, who is in the circle? Serious illness and dying can cause a person's family and community circle to become smaller, but it can also become more meaningful if people put in the work to do so. Often in a person's dying time, there will be family members present, friends, community members, medical professionals, and spiritual support present at different times. It is common to see a decrease in the number of people present as the person transitions further into the dying process. Remember, there is still a lot of work to be done in our culture with people's comfort level with the dying and quite a few people do not want to witness a person pass away. It is not our job as death doulas to force our willingness to be present with the dying onto others; instead, we should strive to be the best example of why it is important to take part in these intense experiences through our everyday presence.

MOVING FORWARD

You have had courageous conversations with the dying and their people and identified their values and wishes in order to build a deathbed ecosystem. What now?

As a death doula, you have many options as to what your

next steps are. You can take the information you have gathered and create a kind of map for your client and those supporting them to reference throughout the dying journey. You can begin to gather resources to provide spiritual or emotional support for your client. You can also begin to build ceremonies or rituals based on what was identified in your conversations with the dying, or you can just show up regularly and be present with the dying person. There is not a defined roadmap of the next steps. What you choose to do depends on you, your skills, and what the person you are working with wants from you. Do not be overwhelmed by the little guidance provided here. What you need to do next is already within you. Take a deep breath, quiet your internal chatter, and really listen for the answers that you already know.

DEATH DOULA STARTER PACK

Now that you have learned about the communication tools and techniques needed to have the conversations necessary to identify what your client wants in their deathbed ecosystem, it is time to begin asking the questions that will help you to map it all out. The deathbed ecosystem consists of what is outside the person – their physical space, what makes their space comfortable to them, who is present with them, and how they want to receive outer physical care. It also consists of what is internal – what emotions they express, their thoughts, unresolved relationship issues, interpersonal interactions, and what supports them mentally and emotionally.

The following questions are meant to be used as a starting point in your conversations with those you serve. They are flexible questions that can change depending on who you are working with and as your doula practice develops. You can move through the line of questions starting with external topics then progressing to internal topics or vice versa. The way you move through them will depend on your conversational flow and the person you are serving's comfort level with the information. Some people will be ready to dig right into the hard questions that have them reflect on their death. Others will need more conversational warm-ups to get to the tougher information. Try different approaches with your clients and see which works best for you – external questions to internal or internal to external.

Communication Energy

To begin, let us discuss a few examples of how the energy in communication presents itself. Preconceived notions, judgments, anxiety, fear, and frustration can create dissonance in the conversation and cause people to close up and not want to share. These break down trust. While genuine openness, non-judgment, and authentic presence can help create harmony and alignment in a conversation by providing a feeling of safety for those in the exchange. These build up trust.

Take a moment to think about how it feels in your body when you experience certain emotions and thoughts. When you are angry, how does it show physically? Does your temperature rise? Maybe your skin reddens? Do you have to tell those around you how you are feeling, or can they tell on their own? Now, think about a recent conversation that you had with someone. How did it go? What was your state of mind during the conversation? What was your emotional state? Did either one affect the way the exchange went?

Continue to practice your noticing skills in your daily life by observing the energy that people bring to conversations and how it affects the experience in order to develop this whole-body observation skill more.

Client Questions

Physical Body

- What does your physical body mean to you?

- What physical issues or illnesses do you live with currently? What are any physical limitations that you live with currently?

- Tell me about a time in your life when you felt the best. What was it about that time that was so good?

- How has your body been cared for during past illnesses or injuries that brought you comfort?

- What things make you uncomfortable or anxious concerning your body in life now?

- What are your daily physical goals?

- Who would you like to care for you physically if you need help? Is there anything particular that they should know about you?

The Room

- Describe where you are most comfortable.

- What physical environment would you like to be in when it is your dying time?

- What bothers you physically – smells, noises, certain light levels, types of fabric, or touch?

- What kind of music or songs would you like to hear, or would you prefer silence?

- What objects, sounds, smells bring you peace and comfort?

- Do you have a favorite blanket, chair, light level, room temperature, etc.?

At the Bedside

- What people from your circles would you like to be with you when you die? Who do you not want to be there?

- Would you prefer a member of your circle relay medical information to you or someone on your medical team?

- Do you have any pets you would like to visit with before your passing?

Medical Changes

- What are you willing to give up in order to live longer?

- How much time for treatment and side effects are you willing to cede in the hope of living a longer life?

- What kind of treatments are you willing or unwilling to have?

- If your family wanted you to take treatments you would rather forgo, how important would it be to take the treatment to keep them happy?

- What bodily changes might make you feel that life is no longer worth living?

Emotional Life

- What are the ten most important things to know about you ranked in the order of importance?

- Describe your emotional life right now? Are you able to openly express emotions?

- Describe any challenges you have with anger, joy, grief, sadness, anxiety, or other feelings?

- Can you share times when you have experienced the emotions listed above?

- What are you feeling most these days?

- What relationships in your life need healing and completion?

- Which relationship would you like to focus on in the time you have left?

- Is there anything disappointing, painful, or incomplete in relationship to your body? If yes, what?

- Have you ever been in a situation that you found intolerable? What made it that way?

- What are you afraid of?

- What have you done in the past when you have been afraid that helped?

- What fears do you have about being in a hospital or nursing home?

- What fears do you have about becoming frail, dependent, alone, out of control, or in pain?

- What fears do you have for your loved ones?

Relationships

- Who are the people you love?

- What are the ten most important things to know about the people you love?

- How might you be able to help them as you die?

- What things do you need to let go of?

- What areas of your life need forgiveness?

- What regrets do you have in your relationships? In your emotional life?

- Can you forgive yourself for anything you regret?

- What relationships in your life need healing and completion?

- Which relationship would you like to focus on in the time you have left?

Legacy

- What has given your life meaning?

- What are you most proud of in your life?

- What is the most important moment in your life?

- What is the theme of your life's story?

- What do you think your most important contribution to the world has been?

- How would your friends describe you? Your family?

- Is there any wisdom that you would like to pass on to others right now?

- What are your favorite passions?

- How would you like to be remembered?

- Is there anything you need to do in order to feel complete?

- Would you like to create a legacy project together? (Videos, writings, photos)

- What objects would you like present with you to entertain, encourage conversations, or spark good memories around you?

- Are there any stories you would like to share with others right now?

Spiritual Life

- Would you like any rituals or nonreligious/ religious ceremonies performed before you die?

- Would you like any poems or prayers read during your dying time?

- Would you be interested in having any singing, drumming, or chanting before you die?

- What other cultural/ spiritual/ religious/ ritualistic practices would you like to be honored with before you die?

Summary Questions

- Summarize your vision for your physical body and your deathbed ecosystem.

- How close is your current reality to the vision for your body and ecosystem?

- What clear steps can we take to move towards your vision for yourself?

7

HANDS ON, HEART OPEN – DEATH DOULA SKILLS

"Where do your beliefs meet your actions?"

— STEPHEN JENKINSON

What is already within you? Something led you to do this work. Something inside of you. One of the most powerful tools to acknowledge as a death doula is that you already have everything you need to do this work within you. We just need to polish it up, give you the confidence to fully embrace your skills, and maybe put a few new practices in place.

In this chapter, we will cover some of the hands-on practices that you can incorporate into your work as a death doula as you begin to move your practices from the head to the heart. This work will start to draw from your inner wisdom as you bring sacredness back to the dying process. Building trust with those that you work with can ease outer and inner pain as we guide dying people home and help those who remain behind find a soft place to land as they are reborn into their lives without their loved one.

What many people want as they enter their dying time is truth, touch, and more time. As a death doula, you can facilitate a way for the truth of the dying process to be shared. You can offer gentle and supportive touch. And while you cannot create more time, you can work with the dying person to distill what should fill up the time they have left.

When sacredness is brought back into the support of a dying person, space for true caring is present. The art involved in being a death doula makes much out of the little time that is left for a person. The softer, hands-on, and heart-open skills that a doula provides create a container for healing relationships, healing presence, a healing deathbed ecosystem, and healing moments during a person's dying time. These skills treat not only the physical aspects of dying but also the soul work necessary to die a good death.

HOLDING SPACE

In order to create a safe deathbed ecosystem where people feel comfortable with being vulnerable and doing the hard work of dying, a death doula must provide a judgment-free container. They must hold space for the people they work with. This means being present physically, mentally, and emotionally for someone in order to focus fully on the person they are supporting and their feelings. It also means that the Doula sets a kind, curious, and open-minded tone for the environment. Holding space is one of the first and easiest ways to connect with and honor the people doulas serve. It is an internal and external act. Put simply, holding space involves deep listening without needing to fix or respond to what is being said, tuning into their own inner knowing and giving those involved permission to do the same, and witnessing the unfolding events from a neutral place. By beginning with the creation of sacred space that respects the dying person's experience and those that surround them, the death doula allows for true expressions of the dying journey to shine through and the opportunity for a good death.

OBSERVE, CONTAIN, FACILITATE

As doulas observe the deathbed ecosystem and all within it, they see what is expressed or held back. Developing skills of a keen noticer allows the doula to see the subtleties felt by all surrounding the dying person. Then they can use their intuition to tune into what is needed in the moment as they work to build a safe environment to contain all the complexities of the dying experience. Doulas also facilitate or fully witness a person's dying time through their actions which teaches the circles of people present to do the same. It is with the looks they give, the gentleness in their voices, and the softness of their touch that death doulas steady a dying person and their people. And it is this steadiness that people need to make it through this experience.

PRESENCE

Presence refers to the way of being with others. As a death doula, this is one of the most vital skills you will employ. It is key to bring a positive and peaceful presence to the dying space. Ways that our behavior demonstrates our presence with the people we serve include allowing for vulnerability and expression of a range of emotions without rushing them, acknowledging that even when someone is dying that their personhood matters, and being sensitive to others by allowing for their individual beliefs and practices while honoring our own.

A sense of presence can also be felt when we embrace

altruistic values and practice loving kindness to others. Death doulas attending the bedside also develop helping, trusting, and healing relationships with those they serve by creating a nurturing environment for the individual's inner and outer realms with respect for human dignity. Doulas share teachings related to the dying experience in a way that addresses individual needs, comprehension styles, language styles. Doulas do this all while being open to the mystery and magic that can enter the dying space.

So, this is a lot to ask of one person to be able to provide this level of interaction with another human. How can one person begin to provide all of this? By starting with ourselves. As practicing death doulas, we must first provide ourselves with all that we hope to give to our clients and it starts with kindness. Begin by treating yourself as you would treat a client you were serving or how you would treat a friend even when things are not as you would wish them to be. Acknowledge the range of emotions that you feel in your life. Allow for the vastness of your lived experience. Show up and be present in your own life for yourself. Only when you do that for yourself, will others truly feel that you are able to present for them.

THERAPEUTIC END-OF-LIFE PLAN

The creation and implementation of a Therapeutic End-of-Life Action Plan is not a medical care action plan. Rather, it is a plan to provide physical comforts outside of the medical realm. This plan can be blended with the medical care plan, but it should not be a substitute for one.

Earlier work of identifying what quality specifically means for an individual and what provides physical comfort during the co-creation of the deathbed ecosystem should be taken into account when creating a Therapeutic End-of-Life

Plan. This plan is co-created with the dying person in mind and brings with it all of the requested comforts along with any healing modalities that you can provide. It takes into consideration the dying person's daily baseline for living, or their starting point, and creates a guide that anyone surrounding the dying person can rely on.

You create this care plan simply by making a written list, a spreadsheet, or a more elaborate document or map to keep on display in the deathbed space. The list can include information that can be utilized when accompanying the dying person such as music preferences, suggested readings, smells that the person likes or dislikes, acceptable T.V. programs to have on, favorite objects such as blankets, to cuddle or not cuddle statements, willingness to receive touch/ massage, etc.

The following sections of the chapter will identify tools and techniques that you can add to the Therapeutic End-of-Life Plan that you co-create with your clients or skills that you can use on an as-needed basis.

PHYSICAL – OUTER BODY SUPPORT

As a person enters into the last stages of the dying process, there are physical supports that the death doula can provide. Preventing skin breakdown or bedsores is important earlier in the dying process when a person is comfortable with being turned and repositioned. Using pillows or blankets, you bump up parts of the body to relieve pressure and prevent skin issues. If the person you are supporting is receiving hospice care, they can guide you on how best to turn or reposition the individual. Otherwise, listen to the person you are caring for and do not position in any manner that brings a great deal of discomfort. Pain can result directly from how a person is positioned in bed. Changing the person's position in bed does not have to be a long-term change, they can move back to their original position after a short period of time.

If the dying person is willing to have someone lie in bed with them and someone in their circle is game to do it, attentive touch and cuddling can provide distracted repositioning of the person. Cuddling or holding can also fulfill the need for a gentle touch. This is dependent upon the prior relationships of the people present; if they openly expressed physical affection before entering their dying journey, then, by all means, it should continue. For some, this is not the case, and a person's dying time can be the first time someone accepts physical affection from some people in their circles. Attentive touch and holding do not always have to be a grand gesture too. Hand holding is an amazing way for people to connect physically that may be less threatening as can be gently touching someone's temple. Read the field of the deathbed ecosystem and encourage physical contact when you feel it is appropriate. It may be that the person you serve is more willing to receive gentle touch from anyone providing medical care or from you. It is also important to advocate for your clients if touch is not requested and it is not something that they are comfortable with.

In life, people often have a comfortable temperature zone for their bodies. What worked for them before will most likely change as they progress through their dying time. Simply identifying early in the planning stages what ways a person likes to be cooled or warmed is helpful especially if they have a preference for fuzzy socks, a specific blanket, or the gentle breeze of an open window. A wonderful way that the circle of people surrounding the dying person can be of support with this is by gifting a special blanket to keep the dying person comfortable. If the space the person you serve doesn't have an efficient heating and cooling system, you can always provide portable heaters or fans as a part of your care.

Other ways to provide outer physical comfort is by offering gentle massage. This does not need to be the deep work of a massage therapist to provide comfort or physical distraction. If you are a trained massage therapist, then utilize your training and skills to the best of your ability to support your client. One of the easiest areas to massage if not a trained professional is by rubbing the dying person's hands gently with their favorite lotion or one of your choosing. If the person you are serving is accepting of it, you can offer light foot or lower leg massage and gentle stroking on the person's back too. It is good to ask those providing medical care to the dying if there is any reason why massage should not be used or if there are any areas to be avoided. Remember to bring the beauty of your nonmedical doula support and blend it with those in the medical circle to best serve your client.

PHYSICAL – INNER BODY SUPPORT

During a person's dying journey, the physical body more readily shows to those present that changes are occurring. What is harder to see is what is taking place in the dying person's inner world. A dying person undergoes a whole host of internal transitions as they begin to release from their physical body. These existential changes can manifest to the outside world as depression, anxiety, apathy, withdrawal, and/ or combative behavior. Death doulas can aid the changes in this less visible realm by implementing nonmedical supports. Often, what is occurring for the dying person cannot be supported by administering a medication; rather, it is an opportunity for the death doula to provide alternative therapies to aid the dying person in the process, or it is a time for the death doula to model acceptance of the changes and work on the act of surrender.

Many times when people find out that they are dying, their reaction is to fight for their lives and find any means to support the battle. This stems partially from our biological need to survive and from our cultural conditioning. Western medicine has many treatments and cures for medical ailments, but it also has its limits. There is no cure for death. What we as death doulas can offer is support as people begin to come to terms with their own mortality.

As a society, we are conditioned by our medical establishment and by our age-phobic culture to push the reality of death off as much as possible. Even traditional doctors are aware of the limits of the human body, but they often cannot suggest withdrawing care for a dying patient because the family of the dying person is not ready to hear that there are no options. The family is not ready to face the idea of death.

It would be easy to place blame for people's reluctance to face death on the medical community, but that is not the case. The root of the phobia is more complicated than that. In fact, relying on blame at all to focus on what is wrong with our death-phobic culture does not help. Blame is not a tool in the death doula's toolkit. Instead, death doulas take time to familiarize themselves with what ails their culture and society along with what ails their clients.

This means while death doulas' work supports one person, it actually begins to heal the whole culture. One of the most beautiful acts you can perform as a death doula is to help the people you serve weave together the traditional medical support they are receiving with alternative therapies. That is healing medicine in itself.

In the following section of the chapter, we will begin to cover some of the non-traditional tools that you can have in your death doula tool kit as you start to see yourself as an instrument of healing during the dying process. The topics covered will include:

- Music
- Reading
- Breath work
- Herbal medicine
- Aromatherapy
- Energy work
- Memory work
- Story building
- Meditation
- Prayer
- Heart-to-heart connection

Music

One way to raise up the dying person is through music. This can be live music or recorded. It really does not matter. Music can provide therapeutic benefits that help alleviate pain, fear, and anxiety. It can provide a beautiful calming distraction that can also help to slow and deepen the dying person's breathing rate. The music should be tailored to what the person you are supporting finds relaxing. This can be a time to bring in sound baths to provide sound healing if your client is open to the idea. The idea behind sound baths is that by listening to tuning forks, Tibetan singing bowls, or other various instruments, stress can be reduced, allowing a person to enter a meditative state of being. This can also facilitate healing which for the dying person can be related to supporting inner healing or soul healing.

Reading

For some people, words can provide healing and relaxation. Reading from religious texts can uplift people and can bring words or reassurance, but readings are not limited to only religious texts. Just like with music selection, what is read aloud to the dying person depends on what brings them comfort. Poems, nonfiction, motivational speeches, hymns, psalms, blessings, mediations all can provide outer relaxation and inner healing.

Breathwork

As we begin discussing breath work, it is important to rely on your own being to establish a baseline in your practice of caring for others. Simply begin by practicing this breath awareness exercise.

Breath Recognition

1. Place one hand lightly on your upper chest and the other on your belly.

2. Take a few breaths in and out.

3. Concentrate on the movement of your hands as you breathe.

4. Note which hand is moving first. Is one hand moving first or are they synchronized?

5. See if you can escort your breath as it moves in and out of your body.

6. Allow your breath to support you as you focus in on its rhythm.

7. Maintain this practice for as long as you would like.

As discussed in Chapter 4, it is very common for people at their dying time to progress through different types of breathing. Receiving care from the person's medical team can support and ease the dying person's struggle with breathing. When a person struggles to breathe, all the organs of the body can be enlisted to help, even the mind. It can be stressful to struggle to breathe. Nonmedical support provided by a doula can help to ease the stress and bring the breathing back to a more manageable state. One simple breathing exercise is synchronizing your breath as you provide gentle hand massage. The intention of this exercise is to audibly encourage a slightly slower and deeper breathing pattern while massaging their hands. This can be beneficial by providing a distraction while offering guidance on breath work. This exercise can provide support at any stage of the dying process.

Synchronized Hand Massage and Breathing

1. First, synchronize your own breathing with your own massage strokes. Breathe in as your hands or fingers move towards your own body. Breathe out as the massage stroke travels in the outward direction.

2. Let the sound of your breathing be slightly audible. A natural interaction will occur, and then with sensitivity, you may find that you can help them relax into a naturally less distressed breathing pattern. This should be done without words, relying entirely on the interactive effect of the combined stroking and breathing. Do not tell the other person to change their breathing, as that will only increase their anxiety, not reduce it.

Match the Breath

Another option is to match the breath of the person you are working with. First, identify their breathing pattern and level of inhalation and exhalation depth. Bring your awareness to your breath and begin to match their rate and depth. Once your breathing matches theirs begin to consciously slow yours while focusing intently on their being. The goal with the matching the breath exercise is to get the person to focus on your breathing rate rather than their own until they unknowingly begin to follow your inhalation and exhalation patterns. This is a good exercise to use earlier in the dying process when the person you are supporting is still alert.

This can also be practiced by placing your hand on the dying person's chest if they consent to it and slowly talking them through your inhalations and exhalations until their breathing pattern returns to a desired state.

Infinity Breath

Begin by breathing in and out. Simply focus your energy and attention onto someone or something that you would like to give to. Bring your breath into an infinity pattern, meaning, breathe in what you need from the world while you breathe out what you would like to give to another. Repeat this practice for as long as desired. Before opening your eyes, do a short three-to-five-count breath-hold to allow yourself to be reborn full of what you needed to draw from the world and what you gifted to the other person.

Exercise 1

1. Take a deep breath from your diaphragm or the muscle between your lungs and belly.

2. Hold the breath for several counts or however long is comfortable for you.

3. Exhale slowly.

4. Place your one hand on your abdomen and the other on the small of your back.

5. As you breathe in and out, allow yourself to release the expectations held in your abdomen. Allow yourself to feel held and safe.

6. Take another breath in and hold for several counts.

7. Let relaxation spread throughout your body as you repeat the pattern for as long as you are comfortable.

8. Upon ending, allow yourself a moment to feel any emotions that came up for you.

Exercise 2

1. Sit comfortably in a quiet space with your gaze lowered or eyes closed and your spine straight.

2. Bring your attention to your breathing. Try to breathe into your belly. Notice it rise and fall.

3. If any thoughts, emotions, physical sensations, or sounds arise as you inhale and exhale, notice them and let them go. Allow them to come and go without judgment.

4. Continue breathing in and out focusing in on breathing into your belly.

5. If you find your mind wandering, notice what took its attention away and then come back to your breathing. Accept any feelings that come without dwelling on them while noticing how your body reacts to any disruptive thoughts.

6. As you finish up your breathing practice, feel free to repeat a phrase or word to keep yourself in the moment such as "forgive" or "calm."

7. Slowly open your eyes and bring your awareness back to your physical space.

Other ways to provide comfort to someone who is experiencing breathing difficulties is to raise the head of the bed or raise up their upper body with pillows. Be aware that you can prevent choking on secretions by positioning the person on their side. The medical team can give medications to reduce moist or rattling breathing sounds. Supplemental oxygen can also be administered to ease discomfort. Remember to provide mouth care in the form of glycerin swabs, moistened washcloths, or sips from a straw if the person is able to swallow to prevent mouth dryness and discomfort.

Herbal Care and Aromatherapy

Herbal care and aromatherapy are options for providing additional support in dealing with symptom relief, lessening stress that accompanies end of life, and supporting grief. Medicinal plants can provide alternative avenues to bring comfort to caregivers, the dying, and the bereaved. A local herbalist may provide you with customized herbal care plans for your clients. As always, this information is not intended as a substitute for medical care. It is important to be aware of any risks involved with combining herbal medicines with traditional medicines.

With knowledge and experience, a death doula can effectively use herbal supports and/ or aromatherapy to provide care to the people that they serve.

Also, alternative therapies do not have to be all or nothing for a death doula. What that means is that based on your experience, comfort level, and knowledge, you can bring any herbs and essential oils that you are willing to work with to your practice. The people that you serve also may have requests for specific herbal allies or essential oils to be used in their dying time. Herbal remedies and aromatherapy can support and aid shifts in perception as they journey through their dying time. They can be especially helpful when dealing with fear and anxiety.

My personal experience with herbal medicine and aromatherapy is limited. What I do use tends to be mainstream such as herbal teas, aromatherapy for the nice smell, salves, and tinctures created by a local herbalist. That does not mean I do not allow myself to rely on these when providing care for my clients. I do use them. It does mean that I do not profess expertise to my clients or you, the reader, in this area. One of the areas that I find most exciting is the research in using cannabinoids (marijuana compounds) and psilocybin (mushrooms) to aid people who are walking toward their death.

Teas

I have found that it is helpful to carry supplies not only to ensure that the dying person is supported but also those surrounding them, including myself. Depending on the location of the deathbed ecosystem, there may already be supplies such as tea and coffee. I pack it along anyway. For me, tea is a talisman. Having it in my bag reassures me that I have something to offer people who need to reset or to be distracted. I also carry hard candies for the same purpose. I use it for my own person when working in challenging situations. You may find that something else works for you. Some of the teas that are recommended to help reduce stress and calm anxiety include:

- Green tea to reduce anxiety (remember it has caffeine, though).

- Passionflower tea to help with sleep quality.

- Lemon balm tea to help with mild to moderate anxiety and insomnia.

- Chamomile tea to help with calm.

- Peppermint tea to soothe the body and calm the mind. Good for calming the stomach.

- Valerian root tea for sleep disorders and insomnia.

- Lavender tea for relieving stress and promoting relaxation.

- Rose tea for a relaxing effect.

- Cinnamon tea to increase warmth.

Flower Essences

I use Bach's Rescue Remedy during intense situations, usually for those surrounding the deathbed. If there is bad news, a family upset or bereavement, feelings of confusion, fear, or any traumatic experience, this remedy will help to face the situation. This is a flower essence that I have used often in my own family and personally. Bach's has an entire line of products, but I am partial to Rescue Remedy Pastille, which is like hard candy, and the Rescue Sleep Melts. The tinctures could easily be used to support the dying person during times of stress.

There are many products available that are similar to Bach's brand. Search for local providers or brands that work for you.

Medical Marijuana

Use varies depending on state laws. Marijuana is still illegal federally, but some states allow for medical use. Medical marijuana use can provide options for end-of-life symptom management that helps to keep the dying person as comfortable as possible. While there are not currently standardized legal forms concerning end-of-life marijuana administration to add to medical records, it should be discussed with the healthcare substitute or agent if the dying person wants to use this form of treatment and if it is a legal option in their community. There are many forms of cannabinoids that can be used. The product does not even have to contain THC, which is the primary component that causes the high associated with marijuana. CBD products can be used without causing a drug-induced high. Consult with a local expert to find out what type of product would best serve the dying person.

Psilocybin and psychedelic drugs are currently being tested in applications for people with advanced-stage cancers and with people who are facing the end of their life. While more research needs to be done in this area, there are promising results that show using psilocybin may be an option for supporting the spiritual side of end of life in the future.

Western culture is beginning to learn what many older, indigenous cultures have known and practiced for generations – that the natural world offers many plant allies when it comes to aiding someone in their end-of-life journey.

Essential Oils

Essential oils are good for diffusing in a room to add a layer of comfort and relaxation for the clients you serve. The oils can also be directly inhaled from the bottle or a couple of drops placed on hands, then rubbed together to heat up the oil and held in front of someone's nose as a carrier to deeply inhale from. As a death doula, you can integrate the use of oils into your practice in multiple applications. Either you can use them based on their recommended uses or you can simply ask your clients to smell a variety of oils and see which ones smell pleasant to them.

Opportunities to use oil include hand massages and anointing ceremonies. I have even left cotton balls with drops of oil on them in plastic containers in a client's room for family members to open up and let their loved ones smell whenever. It can be used as a relaxing agent or a pick-me-up for the dying person and for those surrounding the deathbed. It is important to note, that not all of your clients may be open to using scents in their dying time. It is not uncommon for neurodivergent people to not like strong smells or to not react the same way to the oil as its intended use. As always, how you use essential oils in your practice will depend on your comfort level with them. They are another option available to you. Here is a starter list of essential oils that may work in your practice:

- Pink Grapefruit – a refreshing oil that relieves nervous exhaustion.

- Palmarosa – for those who need to feel love and security, helps to ease emotional upset.

- Ylang Ylang – helps to reunite our emotional and sensual natures, harmonizes the mind and senses.

- Sweet Orange – is a happy oil that uplifts and reduces stress,

• Lemongrass – tones all systems of the body including the nervous, immune, and respiratory.

• Petitgrain – similar to Neroli but has stronger anti-depressant properties.

• Neroli – banishes deep stress and insecurities.

• Bergamot – similar to grapefruit, alleviates stress and elevates mood.

• Peppermint – calming, helps with nausea.

• Lavender – calming encourages sleep.

• Lemon – uplifts mood and helps to relieve stress.

• Frankincense – sacred anointing oil.

• Holy Basil – warming, clarifying, and uplifting; refines mind, body, and spirit.

• Sandlewood – enhances prayer and meditation, calms a busy mind, and reduces worry.

One of the wonderful things about using essential oils is that as humans, we are wired to associate memories with our sense of smell. What that means for you is that you can inquire about smells in your client's life that bring back fond memories such as certain colognes, flowers, or even the smell of clean laundry in addition to using essential oils. Those smells can be used in the deathbed ecosystem to spark conversations or to bring another layer of relaxation to the people you support.

- The use of energy work
- The creation of legacy projects
- Meditation and prayer
- Heart-to-heart connection

Energy Work

Case studies have shown that as a person nears their dying time, the energy field around them changes. Energy medicine deals with two types of fields. One can be measured (veritable energy) and the other has yet to be measured (putative energy or chakras). As a person transitions through the stages of the dying process, the body begins to accept the process, and the energy of the person begins to withdraw until there is a dissipation of the soul.

As a death doula, you can provide techniques to expand the chakras and thin the energy field to enable clearing of what no longer serves the dying person. As the dying person transitions into the active stages of dying, lower-body energy work and touch should be reduced to prevent slowing down the dying process. Doulas can focus on assisting the crown and heart centers to remain open to allow ease in the final stage of dying. The death doula can share energy techniques with the circle of people around the dying person to aid in their dying time.

Many forms of energy work such as acupuncture, healing touch, and Reiki go hand in hand with touch therapies. It is not essential that the death doula be trained in the different modalities of touch therapy or energy work in order to provide support in this area. What is most important is the intention with which the doula interacts with the one they are serving. By working with an open heart and mind, a doula can provide calming energy and peace to a person during their dying time and those in the circle surrounding them.

Reading the energy of the deathbed ecosystem and the person in transition will also alert those in the circle that it is a good time to share stories that they may have never spoken or to give the dying person permission to let go and move on. Usually, there are not big signals alerting those in the circle to energy changes. Instead, it is a subtle energy that can be felt intuitively or by your inner being if you are open to it.

Meditation and Prayer

Buddhist nun and teacher Ven. Sangye Khadro says, "It is said in the Buddhist teaching that helping another person to die with a peaceful, positive state of mind is one of the greatest acts of kindness we can offer." This way of thinking applies to everyone, not only those who are spiritually or religiously inclined. But how can we provide peace and a positive state of mind when a person is facing their death? It comes down to giving the dying person access to something bigger than themselves. Often that can be found in prayer and meditation.

It is important to take into consideration a person's spiritual beliefs when beginning work with meditation and prayer. But in many ways, even those without religious ties can benefit from some aspects of these practices. Practicing meditation with a dying person and the circle of people around them encourages them to focus their attention and possibly shift their awareness.

Praying can be used as a way of communicating with that which is bigger than the individual. Regardless of the name used – God, Source, Allah, Buddha, Creator, etc. – prayer seeks to develop a rapport with the divine. This can have some of the same effects as meditation, refocusing, and shifting thoughts and feelings.

Both prayer and meditation are ways to hand what is being experienced in the dying process over to the universe when seeking support. Even secular people can benefit from the focus, contemplation, and removal from a mind-centered way of being when experiencing distress during their dying time.

Whatever practices you choose to implement will depend on your personal worldview, your cultural background, your spiritual beliefs, and those of the people you serve.

Legacy Projects – Memory Work and Storytelling

As many people enter the pre-active phases of their dying time, they may begin to open up and express a desire to share stories from their life. Ways that a death doula can facilitate this process is by practicing good listening skills and asking deep, curious questions to further the conversation along. Our work with the dying connects them to their past and the stories. Oral storytelling traditions were used by many throughout history as a way to carry meaningful practices and important lessons forward to future generations. Sharing stories with family and friends is a good way to begin expressing how the dying person will be carried forward by their people after they have passed on. Willingness to share memories provides a great opportunity for the death doula to work with the person they are serving to create a legacy project. Creating space for storytelling and shared memories allows the dying person to feel held and heard. This way of supporting someone can lessen the amount of fear they feel around surrendering to death because they know they will not be forgotten.

Options for creating a storytelling and/ or memory legacy project included:

- Memory boxes full of mementos that people in the circles surrounding the dying person can look at together and share thoughts about the objects.

- Recipe books full of commonly cooked foods in the person's life or special occasion recipes. This can be assembled by people other than the dying person and used as prompt to walk down memory lane using food.

- Plaster cast of hands or fingerprints can provide a way for those left behind after a death to physically connect with their loved one.

- Letter writing or video creation can provide the dying person with a way to share valuable lessons or greetings during future special occasions that they would otherwise not be a part of.

- Record the dying person reading children's books for younger generations to enjoy later.

- Assemble photo albums together to provide a conversation starter.

- Create a blanket out of old t-shirts, beloved clothing, or super soft fabric that can be used to cover the dying person or warm anyone else present in the dying space. This can be as simple as buying a premade tie-

> edge fleece blanket from a fabric store or as skilled as sewing a new blanket. My friend Laura Dill, creator of Slay Society Inc., a brain cancer foundation, shared the idea of getting a cheap blanket or sheet and having loved ones write messages of love on it that can then be laid on the dying to person to provide warmth and support from loved ones that may not be able to be present in the dying space.

In my family, one legacy project that I value is my grandfather's writings about and photos from his time serving in the Army Air Corps during WWII. No one prompted him to start writing or sharing stories from his early life. He had never talked openly about it before. Something about being close to his death inspired my grandfather to share as much as he could. It is an amazing gift that my family will keep for generations. This is an example of a self-led legacy project where someone comes up with the idea and executes on their own.

Another experience with a legacy project that left an impression on me was completing a small memory box for a lady entering her dying time. Prior to entering hospice, Linda collected many small, cherished mementos that we placed in a sturdy box that would be kept in near her bed. At first, when people came to visit her, Linda would sort through the box and share memories about the items – a photo of the dance where she met her husband, her children's baby bracelets, a small seashell from a family vacation, a purple ribbon from a hat that she would wear when she went out with her friends, etc. Linda was able to share the stories enough with her family and friends that by the time she was no longer speaking, her people took up the task of reaching in the box, grabbing an object, and sharing the memory with her. Sometimes, they were events that they had taken part in. Other times, only through Linda's storytelling had they become part of the event.

No matter what the project, how big or small, engaging the people you serve in legacy projects provides meaning-based coping for the changes they are experiencing. Creating a project that will outlive them and carry on their memory provides a way for dying people to maintain a sense of self; it allows them to feel pride over their life experiences and to see that their life had meaning. It creates a sense of worth in during a person's dying time.

Heart-to-Heart Connection

> *"And now here is my secret, a very simple secret: it is only with the heart that one can see rightly: what is essential is invisible to the eye."*
>
> — ANTOINE DE SAINT-EXUPÉRY

Heart-to-heart connections with the people you support in your work will look differently depending on the individual. A heart-to-heart connection is seeing the person you are serving for who they are. It is pure, whole-body observation of another human that allows you, the death doula, to connect with their spirit. It means that the roles and responsibilities that the dying person served in life should be acknowledged, but also set gently aside to focus primarily on them as they are now. Once you are ready, you can begin to companion with the dying person and allow space for sacred mysteries such as language changes, non-language forms of communication, and threshold experiences to take place at the end of a person's life.

Companioning

According to Dr. Alan Wolfert's *Companioning the Bereaved,* companioning is a way of being with another person that honors their spirit while not focusing on their intellect or their mind. It starts with your curiosity first and your patience second. When we companion with another, we are not seeking out their expertise; we are seeking to know them as they are, not as the world would have them be. It takes quiet patience and the ability to be grounded in your sense of self to practice. When we practice companioning, we focus on learning instead of teaching, being still instead of full of forward movement while we walk alongside the dying person we are serving. Companioning does not include leading someone to our version of the right answer. It allows us to discover the gifts through gentleness. It asks that we do not fill every unspoken space with words. The words we do use allow those we serve to feel held and secure without providing solutions. It is about bearing witness to the struggles of the dying person without directing those struggles. It is about being present for someone else's pain without trying to fix it or take it away. Companioning is heart-centered and not head-focused. Companioning respectfully recognizes that there is disorder and confusion present in the dying process. While we learn the order and stages of the dying process, companioning does not impose any order on the journey. "Companioning is about going to the wilderness of the soul with another human being. It is not about thinking you are responsible for finding the way out."

The characteristics of companioning are showing empathy, treating others with respect, being warm and caring, and being genuine in your interactions with others. We can practice companionship with gentle words or with sacred silence.

Silent Companionship

Another way to fully be with the people you are serving is by sitting in silence with them. In today's world, people are often uncomfortable with silence. They need to fill every moment with words. By talking over all the silences in the deathbed ecosystem, it is an act of rushing over the moment. People who are uncomfortable in the deathbed space will work to fill their time with words, worrying that they do not have the right thing to say. But when it comes to dying, there is often no right thing to say. The dying process is happening, and it cannot be changed, not with words, not with deeds. A skilled death doula can successfully model how to be silent in the dying space and gently guide those present to release the need to fill the space with words. This does not mean that emotions or words have been repressed during a person's dying time. Instead, this means that opportunities are built into the deathbed ecosystem that allow for the expression of feelings and words that come up along the journey.

By allowing silence to play a part in the deathbed ecosystem, there is space for the unknown to enter. There is space to communicate with the heart. If someone cannot bring themselves to tell a person in their dying time with words how they are feeling or something they have always held back, a silent moment can provide time for them to speak with their heart to the dying person's heart. Quiet moments also allow space to silently meditate and pray. The death doula can facilitate beautiful silent moments during a person's dying time that can provide a healing space for all present.

It is important to adjust expectations of what behavior takes place in the dying space, the expectation of the dying person and of those surrounding the deathbed. As death doulas enter the space of a dying person, they must work to cultivate a deep connection that begins with opening their hearts to that of another. Although as death care providers they may feel a whole host of emotions internally, on the outside they provide a supportive expression of emotion that communicates to the people in the deathbed ecosystem, "You've got this. You can do this. You are not alone." Death doulas follow inner wisdom when providing support for the dying. They take into account their logical minds while leading with a centered heart.

The heart-to-heart connection a death Doula creates with the people they are serving allows them to fully witness the experience. By listening with their heart, doulas are able to lean fully into the moment, validate what is happening for others, and positively regard the experience.

The heart-to-heart skills allow space for the unmeasurable and unspeakable parts of the dying process. This is often the area where experiences happen that cannot be validated by others. It is an area where what is unknown about death looms large. A few otherworldly changes that may occur include changes in the dying person's language that do not make sense in the everyday world, the rise in telepathic communication, and the development of threshold experiences as the dying person balances between the world of the living and what is after.

LANGUAGE OF NONSENSE

As people progress through their dying journey, many changes occur. The way a person interacts with others through the use of language can become less tangible. It can move from speaking with literal language to figurative to nonsensical. Many surrounding the dying person can become disturbed by the changes to what a person says because it no longer makes sense.

Dying people often begin to speak in metaphors and talk about visions and other dimensions that they are experiencing. Phrases and words that come up often in the language of the dying time include:

- Statements of going on a journey
- Seeing visitors and arrival of deceased loved ones
- Needing boxes to carry things
- Metaphors expressing completeness or wholeness
- Announcements of big events
- Repetition
- Narratives that are picked up over several days without prompts
- Mentioning circles to signal unity or completeness
- Expressions of gratitude or resistance
- Words of reassurance
- Numbers, especially three, four, or eight
- Visions of crowds
- Exclamations of motion being felt

ENERGETIC OR TELEPATHIC LANGUAGE

When a person in their dying time begins to speak what some would characterize as nonsense, many often want to correct them or recenter them in reality. It is thought by some that those who are dying have access to truths not available to those who are still fully in the world of the living. Dying people are on the threshold between two worlds and/or multiple dimensions. How can we, who are centered firmly in the world of the living, know fully what it is that they are experiencing? It is possible that as we return to Source, our words and thoughts are elevated by our shift in dimension.

People in the circles surrounding the dying person often feel that they have already lost their loved one when they see language, emotional, personality, and even physical changes even though their loved one is still with them. Remind others to be present with the dying person as they are now. Even with all the changes and losses, the dying person is still themselves.

With language changes, instead of recentering people when they begin to speak of things that we cannot see or are not experiencing, follow their words. Take a moment and enter their world. Let them relive past experiences or talk to long-gone loved ones. It may be difficult for family and friends of the dying person to do this. If you as the death doula explain that it is not an act of relationship diminishment, rather it is a reflection of all that the dying person has lived coming out in the moment, then it may be better tolerated.

Many times, dying people ask questions such as "What is going to happen to me in the days ahead?" "What will happen to me when I die?" "Is there really a God?" or "What if there is really no heaven or God?" No matter the questions asked, it is best to respond by asking another question that will allow the person to guide their own answer. Dying people are carrying an immense emotional load as they are living their deaths. Try not to rush their thought processes, emotions, or the answers that they have within them. They are immersed in the process of releasing from their body, which is full of uncertainty and unknowing.

THRESHOLD EXPERIENCES

> *"As people come close to death, they can begin to start reaching out, as though someone or something is there for them. Language often decreases as hands move in symphony of motion."*
>
> — MARTHA JO ATKINS

Doulas should always act as if the person in their dying time is aware of what is taking place around them and is able to understand voices. It is thought that hearing is the last sense to leave the body. More and more people are beginning to believe that hearing is not the last sense to leave the body; instead, they believe consciousness is the last sense to leave the body.

As a person is progressing through the stages of dying, they sit on the threshold between two worlds – the world of the living and the world of the dead. Dying is an experience that a person lives through that is full of unanswered questions. If we had all the answers to what happens when a person dies, then people would not fear death as much. But we do not have the answers. So, we must allow room for the mystery and magic that appears during the dying time.

One common experience is that visitors come to the dying person. It can be deceased loved ones or angels or other people that they have never met. Either way, it is felt that these visitors come to help usher the dying person on the next part of their journey. These experiences do not need to be validated by anyone outside of the deathbed ecosystem, and those within the space can decide for themselves whether or not anything they witnessed was true or all in their head.

DEATH DOULA STARTER PACK

Forgiveness and Resolving Issues

Unresolved issues, whether they be relationship-based or business-of-life-based, can affect a person's ability to progress through the dying process. They can leave people unsettled and interfere with gaining closure and acceptance. The following practices can be used to aid your clients as they work to resolve matters.

Ho'oponopono Forgiveness Exercise

Thank you for...
Please forgive me for...
I forgive you for...
I love you.
Goodbye.

Ho'oponopono is a Hawaiian practice that corrects, restores, and maintains good relationships among family members and with their gods or God by getting to the causes and sources of trouble. Usually, the most senior member of the family conducts it. He or she gathers the family together. If the family is unable to work through a problem, they turn to a respected outsider. The process begins with prayer. A statement of the problem is made and the transgression discussed. Family members are expected to work problems through and cooperate, not "hold fast to the fault." One or more periods of silence may be taken for reflection on the entanglement of emotions and injuries. Everyone's feelings are acknowledged. Then confession, repentance, and forgiveness take place. Everyone releases (*kala*) each other, letting go. They cut off the past (*'oki*), and together they close the event with a ceremonial feast, called *pani,* which often included eating limu *kala* or *kala* seaweed, symbolic of the release.

This can be adapted to use with honor in your practice as a death doula. Dr. Ira Byock, a palliative care physician and public end-of-life advocate has a similar practice called the Five Final Tasks.

The Five Final Tasks

(From the book *The Four Things That Matter Most* by Dr. Ira Byock)

Will you forgive me? Is there forgiveness that I need from you? Something from long ago? Something that I have carried with me for so long? Can I actually ask for it?

I forgive you. Am I willing to let go of old wounds and hurts in the face of my dying? Let it rest? And can I say it to your face?

Thank you. What a gift it is so say thank you one more time to you.

I love you. This is something we can never say often enough.

Goodbye. Can we actually say it? Let it sink in, this is the final goodbye. Feel all the weight?

8

BUILDING YOUR DEATH DOULA KIT

As you prepare to go out into the world and begin serving people during their dying time, stop and take a moment to reflect on what you have learned so far. At this point, you are beginning to understand that your relationship with yourself is key in your ability to function effectively as a death doula. You have also learned various tools and techniques that you can employ in your work with the dying to cocreate the space they want to die in and ways that those you serve will be carried forward by their people. Now, you will begin to marry the hands-on skills of a death doula and the art of building a deathbed ecosystem with the practical objects needed to perform your work in preparation to support those you serve as they match up what is occurring in their physical world with what is happening in their internal environment through the use of rituals and ceremonies.

In order to prepare to do the work of a death doula, you must first build your Death Doula Kit. Your kit can include a physical bag that you carry around filled with the supplies that will serve your client, the people surrounding them, and yourself. You have to factor yourself into care planning because if your body is not able to function, then you will not effectively be able to serve your clients. Not only does your death doula kit include the tangible objects that you will use in your work with the dying, but it also includes the intangible skills and gifts that you carry inside your person such as conversational abilities, ability to perform energy work, spiritual and religious knowledge, or training in massage therapy. Fill it as full as you wish with physical objects and intangible skills that will aid you as you support the dying, the people surrounding them, and yourself.

DOULA BAG SUPPLIES

Dying can be a labor-intensive process for all involved. Sometimes it can be physically challenging and uncomfortable; other times it can be boring as the people around sit and wait for changes to take place. The supplies you pack in your bag are intended to support the person during their dying journey and after death has occurred. The following list is full of examples of what could be included in your doula bag.

- Your personal comfort care items: phone charger, tea, medications, blanket, shawl, sweater, comfy socks, reading materials, earbuds, money, snacks, gum, water bottle, toiletries, extra underwear, body cleansing wipes, deodorant, toothbrush, etc.

- Emery boards, polish, tweezers, Q Tips, lotion, baby powder, dry shampoo, shampoo caps, comb, brush, etc.

- Oral care for client: mouth swabs, toothbrush, floss,

mouthwash, dry mouth spray, lip balm, coconut oil, denture cleaning tablets, rolled towel, or long gauze to secure mouth closed.

• Eye drops or soft cloth to dampen and place over eyes

• Voice recording app

• Wet wipes, tissues, hand sanitizer,

• Non-latex gloves, face masks

• Bluetooth speaker/ charger, music selections on phone

• Alcohol-free lotions, arnica rubs,

• Guided imagery scripts, white light meditations

• Forgiveness, meditation, joke book

• Spiritual texts, poems, other sacred readings, or any book chosen by client (on your phone, e-Reader, or physical book)

• Anointing Card

• Space cleansing: Himalayan salt lamp, ethically sourced or homegrown herb bundle for smoke cleansing (white sage is used by many, but it is sacred to certain cultures, many other herbs can be used in its place), incense, floral cleansing bowl mixture, matches, lighter (do not use an open flame if client on oxygen), LED candles

• Essential Oils, floral essences, carrier oil, diffuser

• Rescue Remedy, Moxie peace nasal inhaler, hard candies, ginseng or peppermint candy

• Journal, pen, notepad, post-it notes,

• Client file

• Community resource numbers and community guides

• Scissors, tape, safety pins, trash bags, cotton gauze

• Headlamp, flashlight, brown towels

• Singing bowl, drum, maracas

• Camp stool

• MegaMover or portable transport sheet for moving the deceased

• Heavy gloves for dry ice for home funerals

• Bereavement pamphlet, community resource grief list

As you already started to understand in the previous chapters, there is a whole host of practices and skills that you can fill your doula bag with. Many of those skills are beyond my ability to teach you as I am a student in those areas too. Make no mistake, the skills or practices that you do not have experience with are not reasons to prevent you from beginning your work as a death doula. The single biggest gift that we as practitioners offer to help the people we serve is not what we do for them; rather, it is that we are there for them. Being with someone in their dying time is more important than doing for them. All the other gifts we carry in our doula bag are just icing on the cake.

RITUALS AND CEREMONIES

Now that your doula bag is packed to the brim with the tools that will aid you in supporting a person in their dying time, you can begin to take your death doula practice further by supporting the people you serve with rituals and ceremonies.

What do you think of when I mention the word ritual or ceremony? For many people in the Western world, there is a disconnect from taking part in rituals. In our shared history, there has been a time when ceremonies and rituals were considered a punishable offense. Many cultures are trying to regain the loss of these aspects of their societies.

To me, rituals have always seemed reserved for those with deep cultural connections to indigenous and religious practices where they have ways for handling transitioning from adolescence to adulthood, becoming a widow, or death. But for many of us, especially those who lack strong cultural connections, these supporting practices do not feel available. The lack of ritual makes facing significant events, especially death, difficult.

For many of us, ritual practices existed long ago in our heritage, but they have not been passed down or have been long forgotten. The rituals and ceremonies we do practice are often based on the culture of consumerism or have been taken without consent. There are ways to engage in ritual that are not centered around consumerism and do not engage in cultural appropriation. They begin by expanding and developing new models of ritual while consciously honoring cultures who may influence our learning and ritual development. How this applies to the death doula is that you may want to research your own ancestry and see what was available to people in your culture. I do not recommend using another culture's or religion's practices without learning from an expert/ elder from the community.

As death doulas, we can create rituals for the many changes that take place during the dying process, thus providing spiritual care and human connections, even after death. One way that death doulas provide healing for the greater society and culture while serving one individual is through their acknowledgment of the history and experiences they are building their practices on. Two easy ways to implement this into your practice or way of thought is by doing a land acknowledgment and/ or an ancestor acknowledgment. For me, that means I acknowledge that as I write this book in Colorado, I sit on the land that belonged to the Ute, Arapaho, and Cheyenne tribes. I also acknowledge that I am the descendent of some of the first European settlers to North America who had vigorous religious practices and who most likely descended from the native tribes of Britain, Ireland, or Norway. This act of acknowledgment provides me a starting point to research and build my own ritual practices based on my own heritage, my local environment, and what I can learn from the elder cultures in my community while also taking into account my personal spirituality.

As always, death doulas start with themselves. Ask yourself these questions:

- Where are you located?
- Who was the steward of the land you live on before your people arrived?
- What people do you come from?
- What current religious/ spiritual/ cultural practices do you have?
- What traditions did your ancestors carry?
- What cultures are available for you to learn from/ about?
- What practices do you feel you should not use?
- What practices are available to you?
- What rituals/ ceremonies are present in your everyday life?
- What rituals/ ceremonies are present in your life for special occasions?

After you have identified what already exists in your life and what is available to you, you can begin to work on ritual and ceremony creation.

So, what exactly is a ritual? Much of what I have learned about ritual and ceremony creation comes from my teacher, Dr. Sarah Kerr, whom I've already mentioned. I have learned that the simplest way to think of ritual is as an action that has a shared meaning for those participating in the event. They are complex experiences that help people make sense of the event or stage of life that they are going through. They construct meaning on societal and individual levels and they add beauty to our otherwise ordinary everyday existence. Another way to think of it is a *routine* is a pattern that you fall into, while a *ritual* is something that you walk into. Dr. Kerr says, "The structure of ritual can help people rebuild foundations when it has been pulled out from under them."

The death doula's role in end-of-life ritual and ceremony is to be a facilitator for the needed practices and container for all involved. Doulas create a safe space for people to process the personal, emotional, and spiritual changes that occur during the dying journey. They observe what their clients and their people need and create rituals that provide stability and a soft place to land during a tumultuous time of life. Rituals allow a person's soul, their inner being to catch up with what is happening in their outside world.

There are several ways that a death doula can harness the power of ritual to nourish the body and soul of the people that they are serving. Rituals provide a visible container for managing the many changes and losses that occur during the dying process. Before beginning to use ritual, I encourage you to do some research into some of the practices you would like to apply to your work. Learn the history. Work on appreciation, not appropriation, and give credit to the cultures and people you glean your use of ritual from.

THE STRUCTURE OF RITUAL CREATION

Things to consider when creating a ritual:

- Be aware of your state of mind. Maintain a conducive state of mind to what you are creating.

- Keep the people involved in the ritual as the center focus, not the concepts or objects used.

- Although rituals are complex experiences, they can be simple in execution.

- Consider what senses you wish to engage.

- Identify the space where the ritual will be taking place.

- Listen – always listen to what is occurring in the ritual space.

- Be open to surprises. Rituals are living traditions. They move and change according to the situation. Mistakes may be made; new needs may be illuminated during the process. Transitions are difficult.

In creating a ritual, the first step is *identification* of what is needed. As a death doula, you may see that the people in the deathbed ecosystem may need support in dealing with the changes that are taking place. For example, when a person moves from home to assisted living, when the dying person no longer interacts with speech, or when the dying person's breathing pattern changes.

The next step is *preparation*. The death doula must establish the context and goals for the ritual by taking into consideration who will benefit from the ritual. Who are the people, what do they need, and how are they feeling? Consider the space in which the ritual will be taking place. What objects or symbols will be used? What resources are available? Communicate the goals/ intentions of the ritual. The goal of a deathbed ritual is not to fix anything. The goal can be simply a physical act that acknowledges a visible change or part of the transition in the dying process.

Separation follows preparation as those involved in the ritual step out of the everyday mundane world and enter the flexible time period that makes up the ritual. Once people have crossed the threshold into the ritual space, *transformation* begins. After the steps of transformation have taken place, it is time for those present in the ritual space to begin *integration.*

Steps for Creating and Preforming a Ritual

1. Identification of need for ritual

2. Threshold of the ritual – preparation and separation

    a. Approach and preparation
    This time is meant to physically prepare yourself as the facilitator and those whom the ritual is centered upon. This is the time to perform self-care before beginning the ritual and to attend to any needs of the person at the center of the ritual.

    b. Formal beginning or separation
    This time is the start of crossing the threshold where you mark the boundary of the ritual either physically or with words. You enter the actual ritual by creating

and then crossing the non-physical threshold. Everyday mundane life is set aside as the in-between, or liminal space, is entered.

3. Transformation in ritual

a. Orientation
This is the time to set the expectations of the ritual. Communicate the intentions and goals as needed. Let the participants get their bearings.

b. Action
This is where the physical actions, spoken words, or other expressions begin. This constitutes the core transformations of the ritual. Separation from what was known occurs at this point in the ritual. This portion of the ritual can vary in levels of emotional/physical intensity depending on the goals.

c. Release/ reorientation
The key component of the ritual has been performed. Prepare to re-enter the mundane, everyday world. This is the place to begin to regulate emotions and energy levels.

d. Formal closing and grounding
State that the ritual has been completed and the ritual space is being left. State a preparation to return to normality and the everyday world. Take this opportunity to allow people in the ritual to find their feet in their new existence. Allow a practice for self-care and recovery from the ritual.

4. Integration

> a. Decompressing and returning to the everyday
> Reflect personally on what worked and what did not work in the ritual to identify how to deepen the experience next time. Continual practice of ritual is a way to construct identity and build community. Look for ways to provide repeating practices for those present in the deathbed ecosystem to use in their life away from the dying space to help with the transition.

One of the first ways ritual aids the dying process is that it allows those involved to experience death as a collective, communal event. Death is experienced in many ways by the one who is dying as they transition out of their body and by those surrounding the dying person as there is a death of how they relate to the dying person. Even when it is known that death is coming, it is still shocking when it happens. There are many familiar practices to mark the end of life, such as funerals, wakes, and celebrations of life, but there are few commonly practiced ones to mark the process of dying. That is where a death doula can shine and provide something for those in the dying space that they never knew they needed.

By honoring and protecting the dying person and the circle around them with ceremony, we connect to something larger. Many modalities in the western world are about breaking things down to their smallest components or separating things into systems and working on the individual parts instead of the whole. But none of us moves through life alone; even in our individual activities, we exist in a larger system. Viewing our wholeness allows us to own our interconnectedness to those around us. At someone's dying time, viewing wholeness allows those supporting the dying to honor and hold the person's entirety and everything they will lose by dying.

There are layers to honoring and protecting the dying person. Why is the word "protecting" in here? Because performing rituals allows people to embrace the notion that dying is a sacred time of life and that it occurs in a sacred space. It is sacred even if it goes unacknowledged. Sacred objects and events really do not need us to confirm that they are important, but it enriches our experience if we do so. That is where the death doula comes in. The practices in the ritual realm can be performed by you as the doula or you can bring in outside experts to fulfill that role.

TYPES OF RITUALS

Dying Journey Rituals

- Guided meditation
- Prayer
- Vigil
- Creation/ maintenance of sacred space
- Music
- Anointing the dying with shared stories
- Living funerals/ living wakes
- Legacy creation – creating videos, letter, memorabilia boxes

- Story circle
- Deathbed rituals
- Anointing
- Body washing
- Shrouding
- Dressing
- Covering mirrors – old world traditions
- Opening a window as to let the soul out
- Private family mourning space because funerals are often performative and not a good container for grief and processing the loss
- After-death rituals
- Returning to the earth rituals
- Healing and remembrance rituals

One important thing to note is that rituals should be done with intention and thoughtfulness. With this mindset, almost any activity can become a ritual. Remember, a ritual is an action; it is an outside gesture that brings inner meaning. This way of thinking is helpful when working with people that are uncomfortable with the term "ritual" or "ceremony" because you can provide them physical ritual experiences while calling them something else. The gesture is the most important part.

Rituals can be something as simple and as familiar as blowing out birthday candles, having family holiday meals, or something as unknown as drumming a person to their death or washing the body after death. Rituals can be created to meet the needs of the circle.

There are two types of rituals, maintenance rituals and transformational rituals. Maintenance rituals bring people together to more closely connect in communities. Their purpose is to strengthen bonds, deepen connections, and affirm coherence. The type of rituals that live here are birthday celebrations, gestures such as how we greet each other, weddings, christenings, and funerals. The goal is to start the ritual as one person and come out the end of the ritual as more of the same. These rituals are focused on our outer presence and visible changes.

Transformational rituals start with a person going in one way and coming out as something different but in a way that comes closer to your truer self. These rituals included development ceremonies or rites of passage such as those that support moving from childhood to adolescence, adolescence to adulthood, adulthood to elderhood, and elderhood to ancestor.

They attempt to match up the inner world with the outer world.

Examples of Death Doula Ritual Practices

Deathbed Practice

This practice can begin before a person has passed on. Choose songs, poems, and/ or prayers in your preparation work with the dying person to recite or play at the bedside. Read, recite, or play the music while standing at the side of the bed. Take a moment of silence to bring everyone's attention to the process they are witnessing, that they are taking part of, and thank them for their support of the dying and acknowledge the difficulty for both them and the dying person.

Vigil

Vigil simply put is watching over those in their dying time or those who have died. Sitting vigil alleviates the fear of being left alone that some, but not all, express in their dying time. Many cultures and religious traditions have practices for taking part in a vigil. In Western culture, this practice is not as developed, so it may be necessary to inform those not in the immediate deathbed ecosystem what will take place.

The precious hours spent sitting at the bedside of a dying person can be life-changing as it allows people to see the ebb and flow as life leaves the body. Spending time in vigil can also provide the circles surrounding the dying person a beginning to their grieving processes.

Megory Anderson, theologian and the creator of the Sacred Dying Foundation states that "stillness and silence are the cornerstones of sitting vigil."

Another way to facilitate vigil during the dying process is to come together as a family and be with the dying person. It can also be good to allow children and pets to participate if they are willing. The people in the vigil space should work to keep their focus on the dying person, remain calm and centered, and share in the silence. There is flexibility in sitting vigil, and it does not have to remain a silent space. It is dependent on the people present in the deathbed ecosystem and what requests the dying person made.

Vigil can be a time for readings, sharing memories about the dying person, and validating the dying person's experience through words and gentle touch. It may also be a time for reading spiritual texts, singing, or chanting.

Once the person has died, there can be an acknowledgment of the sacred work and duty completed by all those in the dying space by closing out the space with words such as:

> *"South, West, North, and East,*
> *Thank you for holding this space in peace.*
> *Earth below and sky above,*
> *Thank you for holding this space in Love."*
>
> — CHARLOTTE GUSH

After the person has passed away, the circle of people surrounding can remain in vigil and stay present with the body. This is a time for the death doula to gently guide the family and friends in what the next steps are in the removal of the remains and in beginning any requested ceremonies or rituals. This period of sitting with a deceased loved one does not need to be rushed, but you need to understand the guidelines and laws of the area you live in concerning the handling of a dead body.

Story Circle

A story circle can take place at any point in the transition process. The simplest form is during a person's dying journey, those gathered around the bedside engage in story sharing and reminiscing about experiences with their dying. It is uncomplicated and can be facilitated by the death doula by asking questions to those present.

Living Funeral

A living funeral takes place before a person dies, usually when they are alert enough to enjoy the festivities. There is no exact map for how this practice should look. It is a gathering of friends, family, neighbors, colleagues all of whom come together to celebrate a person who is experiencing a life-limiting illness or dying of old age. It acts as a stage for sharing memories, songs, poems, and significant events in the person's life. It is a time to express gratitude for sharing moments of life with the person, to say thank you, I love you, I'll remember you, and goodbye. It allows the whole life of the dying person to be acknowledged instead of just the stage they are in. A living funeral provides an opportunity for the dying person to find renewal in hearing the impact of his/her life.

Giving Permission

Many times when working with dying people, death doulas will experience a stage in the process where it feels appropriate to give the dying permission to complete the work of dying. It is often an instinctive urge felt by someone around the dying person and often comes up when the dying person may be struggling with the ties that bind them to their body. This urge to tell the dying person that can let go can be turned into a small ritual to support the experience by having the loved one gently hold the dying person's hand and say to them, "We love you. Our hearts are filled with love for you. We will never forget you. It is okay to go now."

After Death Options

Moving on to the practical side of caring for the body after a person dies can often be more difficult for people than completing end-of-life paperwork. Both are challenging and both ask the person making decisions to envision what the world will look like while they are actively leaving it or physically gone from it. As a death doula, it is important to be well versed in body care options and even participate in different postmortem procedures.

In most of my early life, the funerals that I attended could be classified as traditional. There was a viewing with an embalmed body in a casket surrounded by flowers. Then came the funeral with eulogies, music, and photos. Then off to the cemetery for the burial in a casket vault. As I got older, I began to experience people being cremated instead of buried. Usually, the funeral was much the same as a traditional embalmed funeral. I even experienced Celebrations of Life – sometimes a party-like atmosphere set up like a carnival or an event much like a funeral only without the deceased's body being present. Another option that I have taken part in is burying cremains in the gravesite of another's. And then there is my mom; her cremains rest on a cabinet in my sister's house where we say she participates in everyday family activities, albeit silently – which is very unlike her. We have still not had an event for her almost eight years after her death.

What I have come to learn is that the options for funerals

are vast. Not even taking into consideration what people of different faiths do, we have countless options for end-of-life ceremonies and rituals. The remaining parts of the chapter will discuss options for the practical after-death care.

Washing, Anointing, and Shrouding

The act of anointing and washing are steeped in historical and ritual heritage. Both can be performed at different stages in a person's dying journey and after they have left their body.

Washing and anointing can be performed as a religious ritual, a secular ritual, or adapted to be performed for those with no religious beliefs. It can be performed as a practice of blessing, of providing protection, refuge, sanctuary, or a final act in preparing the body for disposition. Its power comes from the intimacy of the moment and the touch required to perform it. It is a hands-on experience. Adding an anointing ceremony to your work is a good way to include family in the process if they are willing to participate. It is a practice of connecting one human to another and can be a valuable step in the grieving process.

Water, oil, ashes, smoke, or just the touch of a finger to a forehead can act as the anointing ritual carrier. This ancient practice can be updated and brought into your practice of caring for the dying. How you implement depends on what feels right for you. In the following text, you will find some examples of anointing practices. Use these as they are or adapt them to fit your needs.

Body washing during one's dying journey and after death is one of the most devotional acts of love. Family and friends can be invited to join in on the practice. Many may not want to participate in the entire body washing but may be willing to take part in washing the hands or feet of their loved one.

Bathing can be more than just removing dirt from the body of the person we are serving. In many religions and cultures, body washing or ablutions have potent ritual power and symbolic meaning. It is less about hygiene and more about nourishing the body and soul. It is the physical act of providing spiritual care and human connections even after death.

The washing of the body of our beloved deceased is an ancient and respectful act. In Islam and Judaism, the washing of the body is a common practice. It does not have to be connected with a specific faith or spiritual tradition, as it speaks of an ancient practice that honors the process of connecting with and caring for the body of the deceased in preparation for burial or cremation.

Body Washing

1. Surround the body with absorbent towels or pads. Press on the lower abdomen to remove fluids that may be in the bladder. Have cotton and adult diapers on hand to pack orifices to prevent leakage of bodily fluids.

2. Wash the person's face, gently closing the eyes before beginning, using the soft pad of your fingertip. If you close them and hold them closed for a few minutes following death, they may stay closed on their own. If they do not, close again and place a soft smooth cloth over them. Then place a small soft weight to keep the eyes in position. To make a weight, fill a small plastic bag with dry uncooked rice, lentils, small beans, or seeds.

3. After you have washed the face, close the mouth before the body starts to stiffen. If the mouth will not stay shut, place a rolled-up towel or washcloth under the chin. If this does not

provide enough support to keep the mouth closed, use a lightweight, smooth fabric scarf. Place the middle of the scarf at the top of the head, wrapping each end around the side of the face, under the chin, and up to the top of the head where it can be gently tied. These supports will become unnecessary in a few hours and can be removed. Replace dentures in the mouth if it has been requested.

4. Wash the hair unless it has been washed recently. For a man, you might shave his face if that would be his normal practice.

5. Clean the teeth and mouth. Do not remove dentures because you may have difficulty replacing them as the body stiffens.

6. Clean the body using a face cloth with water and a small amount of soap. Begin with the arms and legs and then move to the front and back of the trunk. You may need someone to help you roll the person to each side to wash the back. If you wish, you can add fragrant oil or flower petals to your rinse water. Dry the part of the body you are working on before moving to another. Some families or cultures may also choose to apply a special lotion, oil, or fragrance to the person's skin.

7. Dress or cover the body according to personal wishes or cultural practices. A shirt or a dress can be cut up the middle of the back from the bottom to just below but not through the neckline or collar. Place the arms into the sleeves first and then slip the neck opening over the head, tucking the sides under the body on each side.

8. Position the arms alongside his or her body or cross over the chest. Be sure the legs are straight. If the person is in a hospital bed with the head raised, lower the head of the bed to the flat position. Place ice packs or dry ice around the body under decorative blankets or pillows if the temperature is hot or if the body will remain in place for a longer period.

Before beginning either anointing or body washing, make sure you have grounded yourself. Take time to meditate or set aside any thoughts or distractions you have that could interfere with the process. You can begin by partaking in a purifying process for yourself before your start. Also, remember to set your intentions for why you are performing this ritual. There is no right or wrong way to perform these ceremonies as long as the intention behind comes from a place of love and respect. Both practices can have profound effects for all involved. It is also important to note that participation in these practices is optional for those in the circles surrounding the dying person.

Anointing

Sacred Passage Doula Anointing Ritual Script

(From Conscious Dying Institute)

This script can be individualized as needed. Use soft lighting and soft background music. Use an essential oil such as lavender or frankincense or another carrier oil. Place a drop of oil with a thumb at each body part while saying:

Forehead: We anoint this body, may (name) rest in peace.

Eyes: We anoint these eyes that have seen so much. May (name) rest in peace.

Mouth: We anoint this mouth that has spoken truth and love. May (name) rest in peace.

Shoulders: We anoint these shoulders that have borne many burdens. May (name) rest in peace.

Heart: We anoint this heart that has loved so well. May (name) rest in peace.

Hands: We anoint these hands that have worked so hard. May (name) rest in peace.

Feet: We anoint these feet that have traveled so far. May (name) rest in peace.

Sacred Dying Anointing

(Adapted from Megory Anderson from the book Sacred Dying, Creating Rituals for Embracing the End of Life.)

This is a good practice to do as a group. Take oil and say a blessing over it. One person starts with the forehead and speaks then passes it on to the next person to repeat on a different body part and then on to the next person.

Place drops of oil using your thumb over the areas of the body as you repeat these words:

Forehead: (Name), may this oil heal your mind from all worries and fears.

Hands: May this oil heal you so you can use your hands again in blessing and good work.

Feet: (Name), may this oil heal you so you can walk down your path, whether it be in life or in death.

Heart or over wounds: May this oil heal your brokenness and your pain, and may it give you strength in your heart.

Shrouding

A shroud is a large cloth made of a variety of materials wrapped around a corpse for protection, utility, and/ or spiritual reverence in preparation for burial or cremation. Different cultures create burial shrouds from cloth, animal skin, or plants like bamboo. They are almost always created from natural fibers. Shrouds can be handmade or bought from a store. The materials used are most often biodegradable and will allow the body to decay after burial, but sometimes they can naturally preserve the body. Many cultures have shrouding practices still in use today, and shrouding is regaining popularity in the green burial movement. The act of shrouding is the last way to connect and protect a loved one before returning them to the earth. It is an act similar to swaddling a baby to ensure that the baby feels held and safe. Here are two examples of how to use shrouds:

Shroud with Handles

1. Unfold the shroud onto a clean dressing table. Make sure that the area is clean, as the shroud may drape over the sides and touch the floor.

2. Flip the shroud over so that the pouch is facing up and the handles are facing the floor. If you are placing the shroud into a casket or onto a carrier, skip ahead to Step 4.

3. If using a board, insert the tapered end into the pouch first and slide board into desired location.

4. Place the body onto the shroud. If using a board, center the body on the board. To correctly support the body weight, position the board between the back of the ankle and the top of the neck.

5. Fold shroud over feet to wrap the feet.

6. Cover the body, starting on one side and diagonally folding the corner from foot to the opposite shoulder, and then from shoulder to the opposite foot.

7. Repeat Step 6 for the opposite side of the body.

8. Fold the end down over the head.

9. Fold the sides inward over the body.

10. Gently yet securely fasten the ties into a bow.

11. Decorate the shroud if you wish.

12. To move the shroud, lift by the handles. *Do not drag.* Dragging can cause the fabric to tear.

13. To transport the shrouded body in a vehicle, we recommend that you use a casket, willow carrier, gurney, or stretcher.

Shroud with No Handles

1. Unfold the shroud onto a clean dressing table. Make sure that the surroundings are clean, as the shroud may drape onto the floor.

2. Flip the burial shroud over so that the hemmed edges face upward, then place the body onto the shroud.

3. Fold shroud over feet in order to wrap the feet.

4. Cover the body by starting on one side and diagonally folding the corner from foot to the opposite shoulder. Then fold from shoulder to the opposite foot.

5. Repeat Step 4 on the opposite side of the body.

6. Fold the end down over the head.

7. Fold the sides in and over the body.

8. Slide ties beneath the shrouded body.

9. Gently yet securely fasten the ties into a bow.

10. Decorate the shroud if you wish.

11. Because the burial shroud is simply a wrap and does not have handles or support, you should use it inside a casket or willow carrier.

Alternative to Shrouding Options – Private Mourning Space Rituals

Option 1

For those who you serve who do not wish to be shrouded, one way the family and people around the deceased person can participate in one final more intimate act with their loved one is the practice of covering and speaking words. To prepare for this ceremony, make sure the decedent appears comfortably positioned in bed, hands resting at sides (under the blanket may be easier, but I like to leave hands out for people to hold and touch). Have a sheet or light blanket over the deceased's body that will be able to be brought up over their face at the end of the ceremony. Prior to starting the ceremony, make sure that one person is designated as the last person to speak and cover the body. This is a good discussion to have on the choice of who this should be during the end-of-life preparations. Gather everyone around the deathbed. Those who wish to speak can share a statement of gratitude and/ or release one at a time until the designation person speaks last and then brings the sheet up over the face of their loved one to signify that the next part of the dying journey has started and everyone can begin grieving.

Option 2

After someone passes away and is removed from their deathbed, especially if the death takes place somewhere other than a medical facility, it is hard for the people left behind to see the empty, disheveled room. The death doula can ease this experience by preparing the room. Simply remake the bed with fresh linens if possible, dim the lights, open the windows to let in fresh air if an option, and place a single flower on the head of the bed while the funeral director or whoever is transporting the body is readying the body for removal.

Small, thoughtful steps such as these will help to leave positive impressions on those left behind after a death, even if they do not choose to engage in rituals or ceremonies. Remember, not everyone that you will serve will be willing to go all-in with the many offerings you provide as a death doula. The acts of human connection that you build and facilitate are part of the reason that your work heals society as a whole.

Returning the Body: Funerals, Cremations, and Such

The options for how to return the body back to the earth are diverse. Depending on where the person you serve lives and what their wishes are, many ideas for how a person can be returned or reconnected to the earth can be fulfilled. Many times, what a person desires to have happen to their body depends greatly on their values in life. The death doula can work to help the client understand what options are available to them and identify what aligns with their values. This chapter includes a rundown on the options available for the disposition of the body after death. It is important for the death doula to stay educated on what is available in their community and possibly advocate for more options if the community desires it.

There are many more terms and pieces of information that can be learned in regards to handling of deceased remains. All of the methods of disposal come with their own language and processes. It is important as a death doula to have a general understanding of what options are currently available in your area. Death doulas can also work as educators and advocates, informing their communities on what the possibilities exist for after-death care and working to bring different practices to their regions.

Home Funeral

Death doulas can help organize a home funeral and act as a guide during the ceremony. In most states, it is legal to keep the decedent at home until time to transport for cremation or burial. In most cases after an expected death, family and friends can stay with the body for a period of time before contacting a funeral provider for removal. Home funerals can save money by bypassing traditional funeral expenses, but the family of the deceased must be fully willing to participate in this type of service. While home funerals are becoming more common, the practice is not widely accepted. Coffins, baskets, caskets, and shrouds can be made or purchased for the funeral. If a home funeral is desired, investigate local laws and requirements to ensure it is permissible. A home funeral consultant can be hired. Some states require hiring a funeral director even for home funerals. Authorities need to be contacted even when a home funeral takes place to file a death certificate.

Home funerals allow people the privilege and responsibility of taking charge when it comes to managing death care within our own communities. It offers a beautiful and healing experience for loved ones and may be more affordable and respectful to the environment than contemporary funeral industry-led funerals. At present, families can take care of everything that is necessary on their own without hiring a funeral director in forty-one states. In the other nine states (*NY, NJ, NE, IL, FL, LA, MI, IN, CT, IA*), the laws may require hiring a funeral director to provide specific services including filling out paperwork and transportation of the body. Hands-on care is still an option for families if that is desired. It is important to consult local laws concerning home funerals and learn when to utilize outside experts to get death certificates.

At one point in time, every funeral was a home funeral out of necessity. Now, we have multiple options of where funerals or memorial services can take place. Many people are returning to having funerals at home where the deceased was most comfortable. There are many factors that need to take place to ensure a home funeral is done properly. A death doula can act a guide during this time in supporting the people left behind as they take a more hands-on approach to returning their loved one to the Earth.

Basic Steps in Home Funeral Planning

- Prepare, wash, and dress the body
- Make the necessary arrangements to move the body
- Arrange for a casket, shroud, or urn

• Keep the room cool

• Obtain ice packs from a funeral home or dry ice to keep the body cool and absorbent pads to collect any fluids.

• Organize the details of the service

• Arrange for burial or cremation

• Complete the paperwork required by the vital statistics agency in your province or territory. This commonly includes the registration of death, medical certificate of death, and burial permit.

Traditional burial

The most traditional burial choice, in-ground burial, typically involves a casket and is marked by a memorial tribute. Below-ground burials usually are contained in a vault or a concrete enclosure to ensure the ground above the casket does not shift. Some states require vaults.

Green burial

A way of caring for the dead with minimal environmental impact that aids in the conservation of natural resources, reduction of carbon emissions, protection of worker health, and the restoration and/ or preservation of habitat. Green burial necessitates the use of non-toxic and biodegradable materials, such as caskets, shrouds, and urns. "Green burial" refers to this process but also to the cemetery in which the burial takes place. A "green cemetery" uses no artificial pesticides and none of the bodies buried in a green cemetery can have been embalmed or buried in a traditional casket.

Natural Burial

A natural burial does not use embalming fluid, a casket, or a burial vault. Instead, the remains are placed directly into the earth, allowing the body to decompose naturally. The process has a minimal impact on the environment. In some instances, the bodies of the deceased are buried in a biodegradable casket or a simple burial shroud so long as they do not inhibit the decomposition of the body in any way. Natural burials also do not use any machinery or heavy equipment for digging the gravesite. Instead, the gravesites are dug manually. "Natural burial" strictly refers to the actual burial process. This means the opening and closing of the grave, the preparation of the remains, and the laying of those remains in the burial plot.

Composting Funeral

Human composting, also called "natural organic reduction," is thought to be a much greener and energy-efficient way of disposing of our remains. Companies such as Return Home and Recompose use a method that works by entombing the body in a capsule filled with wood chips, alfalfa, and straw, along with bacteria that love to chow on organic matter. Dressing the remains in compostable garments such as Coieo burial suits or clothing designs by Pia Interlandi also add to the body's ability to quickly to return to the earth.

Burial at Sea

The United States Environmental Protection Agency allows burial at sea in ocean waters. Human remains need to be placed into ocean water three nautical miles from shore.

Direct Burial

Direct burial is a burial option in which the body is buried within the several days immediately following death, without a memorial or formal funeral service. It is a popular option because it allows people to avoid many of the higher costs associated with traditional funerals and memorials.

Celebration of Life

A celebration of life is an alternative to a funeral. It is an event that focuses primarily on the life a loved one lived, and the legacy that they leave behind. Sometimes even with a party-like atmosphere, a celebration of life tends to be just that – a celebration. The focus is on happy memories of the deceased rather than on the sad fact that they're no longer with us.

Wake

A wake is a social gathering associated with death, usually held before a funeral. Traditionally, a wake takes place in the house of the deceased with the body present; however, modern wakes are often performed at a funeral home or another convenient location. It can be held in place of a funeral as a social celebration of the person's life.

Viewing

A viewing is the time that the family and friends come to see the deceased after they have been prepared by a funeral home.

Cremation

Cremation is the process of reducing a dead body to mostly tiny bits of bone resembling ash that involves exposing the body to flame and intense heat followed by pulverization of bone fragments.

Witnessed Cremation

Witnessed cremation allows the family to watch as the body is brought into the cremation retort and the process of cremation is begun. Viewers will not see the flames but rather see the casket or container being placed in the retort. The entire process can take two to three hours plus the time needed to allow the cremation chamber to cool. There are no laws regulating viewing cremations. Rules and procedures for witnessed cremations are set up by individual facilities.

Open-Air Cremation

Open-air cremation involves burning the body of the deceased on a funeral pyre outside.

Crestone, Colorado is currently the location of the only outdoor human cremation facility in the United States, although Maine is working to pass laws approving the use of outdoor pyres. The funeral pyre is perhaps best connected in culture by references to the ancient Vikings. It is still a death ritual practiced today amongst Buddhist and Hindu religions.

Direct Cremation

Direct cremation is a disposition option in which the body is cremated in the days immediately following the death without a funeral service beforehand.

Water Cremation

Water cremation/ alkaline hydrolysis is also called aquamation, biocremation, resomation, or flameless cremation. Alkaline hydrolysis is a process for the disposal of human and pet remains that uses a solution of 95 percent water and 5 percent potassium hydroxide or sodium hydroxide to reduce a body to components of liquid and bone. Bone fragments are collected, dried, and turned into a substance similar to cremated ashes. The bone byproduct of water cremation may be scattered, buried, or disposed of in any way cremated ashes are handled.

The liquid byproduct of alkaline hydrolysis is a nontoxic solution of amino acids, peptides, sugars, and soap that can be disposed of through local sewage systems. Essentially, alkaline hydrolysis mirrors the chemical decomposition that happens when a body is buried, except water cremation takes just hours, from three to twelve depending on the temperature and pressure in the chamber instead of months or years.

Scattering Ashes

Scattering ashes involves just that – spreading cremains in nature. Officially, permission should be requested before scattering ashes on federal land. However, you will probably encounter no resistance if you conduct the scattering ceremony quietly and keep the ashes well away from trails, roads, facilities, and waterways. You can find guidelines for scattering ashes on the websites for some national parks. The federal Clean Water Act requires that cremated remains be scattered at least three nautical miles from land. If the container will not easily decompose, you must dispose of it separately. The EPA does not permit scattering at beaches or in wading pools by the sea. Finally, you must notify the EPA within thirty days of scattering ashes at sea. The Clean Water Act also governs scattering in inland waters such as rivers or lakes. For inland water burial, you may be legally required to obtain a permit from the state agency that manages the waterway. Scattering by air is limited in that federal law prohibits dropping any objects that might injure people or harm property. The U.S. government does not consider cremains to be hazardous material. So all should be well as long as you remove the ashes from their container before scattering. As always, check local laws and with local authorities before scattering any remains.

Planting Ashes

On their own, cremation ashes are harmful when placed in or around plants (https://letyourlovegrow.com/blogs/blog/why-burying-ashes-is-harmful-to-the-environment). When cremation ashes are buried directly into the ground, they do not decompose, which hurts the surrounding plant life. For cremation ashes to become beneficial to plant life, the very high pH level has to be lowered, and the toxic levels of sodium must be diluted. Products like "Let Your Love Grow" can be added to ashes to bring them to levels that better serve the soil. The Living Urn can be planted with a tree to grow a memorial tree.

Other Options for Ashes

Ashes can be pressed into a diamond; they can infuse a portion of cremated ashes into a glass decorative piece. They can be added to jewelry. Ashes can be mixed with ink to create a memorial tattoo. Ashes can be scattered at a special place with a biodegradable scattering urn (https://www.thelivingurn.com/products/eco-scattering-urns), buried in a bamboo burial urn (https://www.thelivingurn.com/products/eco-burial-urns). The ashes can be formed into stone-like solids. Every day, more options are available for ways to memorialize cremated remains.

Embalming

Embalming is the process of preserving a body to delay the natural breakdown of cells, which begins when they die. It temporarily helps prevent the processes that cause our bodies to decay. It's a funeral practice (https://www.funeralguide.co.uk/help-resources/arranging-a-funeral/arranging-a-funeral) that's been carried out for thousands of years in one form or another. In its modern form, it's been widely practiced since the early twenties. Embalming became widely used in the United States during the Civil War as a way to transport soldiers killed in battle back to their homes. Jewish and Muslim funerals prohibit embalming the body. Depending on environmental conditions, climate, moisture in the soil, and the type of coffin a body was buried in, it can take between eight to twelve years for an un-embalmed body buried six feet down to decompose to a skeleton. While embalming slows the process of decomposition, it does not prevent it altogether. Embalming fluids are generally formaldehyde-based and can adversely affect the environment and have health impacts. Embalming is not known to have any environmental or health benefits and is only rarely required by law, such as in some instances of interstate transport of the remains or following death by infectious disease. Contrary to popular belief, an un-embalmed body will not spread disease in the surrounding environment, according to the Center for Disease Control. There are options for green embalming which uses biodegradable, non-toxic, non-carcinogenic, and formaldehyde-free alternatives to conventional embalming fluid. The process of embalming is the same regardless of which fluid is used.

Whole-Body Donation

Whole-body donation is the process of gifting remains after death to an organization that used human bodies in research such as medical schools, universities, and other research institutions. It is a wonderful way to create a lasting legacy by supporting learning and necessary research. Whole-body donation is complicated because there is no single organization or network that oversees the process of matching donors with research programs and medical schools. Donating your body to science is not the same as being an organ donor (https://www.pcrm.org/ethical-science/animal-testing-and-alternatives/human-tissue-research). The steps needed to become a whole-body donor depend on the state of residence or what type of program desired to donate to. Some states have state anatomical boards (https://ieds.online/body-donation-programs-by-state/) to contact to step up donations. In other states, the receiving institutions must be contacted to see the qualifications for their body donation programs. The organ donor designation symbol on the back of a driver's license does not imply consent for whole body donation. A whole-body donor would need to register with the whole-body donation organization before death. Donating is an extremely time-sensitive process, so it is important to talk to loved ones and make sure they are aware of after-death preferences. Many whole-body donation programs offer services at no cost to the donor or the donor's family. The organization that receives your gift may cover the transportation and cremation costs related to the donation process. Make sure you talk to the organization about any costs associated with the end of life.

Organ Donation

For someone to become an organ donor, they have to die in very specific circumstances. Not every death qualifies to be an organ donation. Most often, a person dies in the hospital because of illness or accident, such as severe head trauma, a brain aneurysm, or stroke. The person is put on mechanical support, which keeps blood with oxygen flowing to the organs. More often than not, after death, a person will be ineligible to donate organs due to the cause of their death, but they may be eligible to donate tissues and bones. Speaking with the medical care team about a person's options to donate is the best place to start the process of gifting tissue and bone.

Healing and Remembrance Ceremonies

These types of ceremonies can occur at set points in time that were decided upon during the end-of-life planning work or can be created on an as-needed basis. Sometimes in your work as a doula, you will help people that experienced a loss in the past they have not come to terms with. The creation of a ceremony that honors their current state of being and their loss can help them to begin a new chapter in their grieving process.

When your work with a client during their end-of-life planning creates a timeline for remembrance ceremonies, you can create them based on the input received from the dying person you worked with, the time frame that has passed, what the people left behind still need, cultural traditions that honor the grieving process, or whatever you see that is needed.

These types of ceremonies are a great way to honor the grief that is felt after time has passed by the people left behind, as they may still need ways to embody the experience. They are also helpful because the community often moves on much faster after a death than those closest to the one that has died. These practices give the inner being, or the soul, time to catch up to what has happened in the external world.

DEATH DOULA STARTER PACK

In working as a death doula, people develop firm thoughts on what practices should take place or be utilized in after-death care that aligns with their living values. Circumstances may arise when a person that the doula serves does not have the same ideas on what should take place after death as the doula. When there is an incongruence of beliefs, either the doula can decide to hold their beliefs in their heart while serving the beliefs of another, or it can become clear that the client and the death doula are not a good match for each other. Not being a match is okay because sometimes the dying want to be served by people that can provide specific religious components or belief systems that your work does not offer. Sometimes the best way to serve someone is to refer them to someone who is a better fit for them.

It is important to understand and own the fact that although we as death doulas feel that our work serves every person, not every person wants to be served by us. By beginning to realize that our work serves people even when we are not directly working with them in their dying, we begin to own the power in our profession. Your training, knowledge, and experience improve the dying experience for all people, not just those you work with.

Client Questions

Spiritual Life

- How do you define Spirit?

- If any, what religion do you practice?

- What are your beliefs about the afterlife?

- If you have no religious belief or spiritual ties, what ways do you like to mark significant events in your life?

- What are the ten most important things to know about your spiritual/ internal life ranked in the order of importance?

- Which of your loved ones might be waiting for you after you die?

- What, if any, spiritual guides or figures may be there for you?

• Have you imagined a place where you will go after you die, where you will rest and be in peace?

• Would you like to be anointed? During your dying process? After death?

• Would you like a body washing ceremony?

• Who would you like to help with body washing? Who do you not want there?

• How long would you like your body to be left in place before removal for burial, cremation, etc.?

• How would you like your body cared for prior to any ceremony or funeral – embalming, dressed up in certain clothing, make-up, etc.?

• Do you want a deathbed vigil? For how long and who would you like it to be open to?

• Do you know what your options are for end-of-life body disposition?

• What type of funeral, ceremony, witnessed cremation, or celebration would you like?

• Where would you like the funeral, ceremony, or celebration to take place? Has it been arranged already?

• What types of care have you heard of outside of your traditional realm of after-death care that you might like to incorporate into your plan?

- What are the ten most important things to know about your after-death care wishes ranked in the order of importance?

- What kind of music or songs would you like to have at your end-of-life ceremony?

- Who would you like to facilitate your end-of-life ceremony?

- Who would you like to speak, perform, or doing a reading at your ceremony?

- Would you like to incorporate food or feasting into any of your ceremonies?

Summary Questions

- Summarize your vision for any end-of-life ceremonies you would like to have.

- How close is your current planning to the vision?

- What clear steps can you take to move towards your vision for yourself?

9

OWNERSHIP AT THE END

How do we allow for ownership at the end of life? How do we empower those who are providing care to a dying person and those whose dying time has come? How do we empower ourselves to walk into the dying space and offer ourselves fully to the experience? Where will the confidence you will need to perform your work come from?

One way we can provide ownership is by allowing ourselves to be fully present and open to what is in front of us. This means to know that we walk into the dying process not to have all the right answers, but to bring willingness to be with people during intense and sometimes painful situations. Our ability to be present applies to the people providing care – those surrounding the dying, as well as those who are actively dying. For each party, the experience may look and feel slightly different, but it starts with the same premise: giving yourself permission to own your wishes and the values held dear that will carry you through the end of life.

OWNING DEATH

Western culture does not often provide a means for us to look at the many levels that we experienced death and dying through. It sets us up to look at it from the materialistic perspective – that death consists mostly of lists of possessions to organize, medical and legal forms to authorize, and physical losses to experience when, in fact, our death involves so much more.

Our current model for handling and supporting death does not provide for the changes a person's soul undergoes or for the changes to their community. It attempts to hurry grief along while not permitting us to live like we are mortal creatures. In other words, we must rush through our feelings after losing someone dear to us while pretending death will never come for us. But, as I've said, death is 100 percent fatal for 100 percent of the population. We will all die, and that cannot be changed. However, the model of care that we provide to our community can be changed. That is where you, acting as a death doula, come in. The attitude that our culture carries about death can either give us freedom in the experience or make us feel powerless.

One of my favorite teachers, Stephen Jenkinson, founder of Orphan Wisdom School, held a potted plant up at a hospice conference once and asked everyone present to describe what they saw. People began to state the obvious, that it was a plant. What they were missing was the decomposition that takes place in the soil in order for the plant to grow. Something has to die in order for other things to grow. We can think about the literal aspects of death replenishing the soil and providing nutrients for the new growth. We can also refer to the figurative aspects of this; how a person dies – not what they die of – will affect the relationships left behind. It will leave a lasting impact on the people involved in the experience.

> *"All the deaths of all living things feed life: what does our death feed? All of life's deaths mean that life continues; what does our death mean?"*
>
> — STEPHEN JENKINSON

The way we live our deaths, the way we communicate about our dying time, and the way we involve those who are dear to us nourish and educate those we leave behind. How do you want to feed the world when you are gone? How do you want to feed the world while you are still physically in it? Through both parts of life – living and dying – we can work to shape the world as we would like it to be. If things go as they should, I will leave this earth before my two children. Being gone means that I will not be here to care for them as I would want them to be when their dying time comes. For me to leave this world knowing my children will be cared for as I would care for them, I have taken a step in creating the world as I would like it to be by teaching others how to care for people in their dying time. By teaching you, my dear reader, how to wholeheartedly provide support and guidance in your communities, it touches my own community.

The art of working as a death doula means that you recognize that the death of one person is much more than just one person leaving their physical body. It impacts the circles of people surrounding the dying person, it affects those who enter the circle to provide care, it affects the greater world because giving one person access to die a good death gives us all access to the same experience. There is death and rebirth in the dying process. The people left behind have to be reborn into their new lives where their loved one is no longer physically present. They have to reform a relationship with the person they lost because even though a person is physically gone from this planet, the relationship doesn't stop; it is transformed.

It is through your work that the people in your community will begin to see a new model of care, support, and relationship with the dying during their dying process and beyond. That is a big thing to carry, but carry it you will.

By working with a death doula, people will be able to hone in on what their wants and wishes are while aligning the end of their life with their values. They will be able to say how they want to feed the world when they are physically gone from it and how they want to be carried by those they leave behind. You will help to build a safe place to allow their work to blossom. You will not provide them with the answers, but you will give them back some of the power that was taken away from them when they learned they were dying.

Completing end-of-life preparation work, the forms, the lists, and practical tasks of mapping out their deathbed ecosystem are key parts to alleviating any mental strains during a person's dying time. The early work of end-of-life planning that is completed with the help of lawyers, medical professionals, and possibly death doulas done by a dying person can help weed out any distractions that could prevent a peaceful transition. Some death doulas choose to support their clients in the paperwork process; others do not. Whatever you choose to do in your practice, it is important to advocate that your clients take the steps necessary to complete the legal and medical paperwork with someone. Having the awareness of what will happen to the material possessions and worldly responsibilities takes some of the pressure off of the dying person. Completing the paperwork also ensures that your client's medical and legal wishes can be fulfilled. Doing this allows the dying to relax instead of worrying about the material world and do the soul work necessary to let go of the attachments to life peacefully because it is our job not to fix the fact that a person is dying but to prepare them and support them in the process. Breathe in the fact that your work will create a safe, secure place where the dying person can fully own what they are experiencing, even when they are no longer in control.

OWNING YOUR WORK

Every death you support, every lesson you learn, every book you read, conversation you have about death and dying will further your embodiment – your ownership of your art. This is not a job that will look the same every day. The skills that you bring to your work will change. You will learn to identify and adapt to what is needed in the moment without losing who you are.

It is my opinion that everyone should receive the support of a death doula in their dying time, but I can tell you from experience that not everyone wants the support we offer. We cannot force our work onto people. It is not in the nature of a death doula to do so anyway. What we can recognize is that although we are willing to work with anyone and everyone, not everyone wants us. Even the people that would like the support a death doula provides may not match with you individually. Usually, people are hesitant to work with a doula because they lack understanding of what it is that doulas provide. This is where your ability to communicate specifics about the services you provide, your ability or inability to support specific faith traditions, and your willingness to work within boundaries that make the dying person comfortable is important. It will be through your words that you will reach their logical mind and with your presence that the person you are working with will connect with something in you that makes them feel safe. It will be almost unknowable to them when a connection is made. Death doulas embody the principles of their work so deeply that what they do is often unexplainable to the mind while being clearly felt by the heart.

Begin to own that you can provide this for others. To do that, you can organize the necessary material and practical steps to support a dying person and the circles that surround them. You can build a container that respectfully allows the dying experience to unfold, and you facilitate rituals and needed practices that fully support people during a deeply felt transition.

OWNING THE WAY FORWARD IN BUSINESS

When the time comes for you to begin working as a death doula, you have many options. In some communities, practitioners such as doulas are already accepted and utilized by the people residing there. It is not uncommon, though, to have communities where the work that a doula provides is unknown. If the geographical area that you hope to serve does not have alternative practitioners working in the community and you may be the first to start serving them in this way, it could seem overwhelming. At one point in time, therapists were not widely known about, and even when there was awareness, working with one was not readily accepted behavior. Even today, many areas do not have proper access to mental healthcare. A practicing death doula can fill in some of those gaps by providing soul care to their community during dying journeys.

Before setting out to provide support to the dying in your community, it will serve well to identify which type of community yours is and to find areas where your services can best serve your neighbors.

Identifying potential businesses and residential homes that you can connect with to develop a working relationship will help you reach more people. Reaching more people means that you will be able to support more people during their dying time. If people do not know that your services exist, then they will not come to you for help. Practicing doulas do have to make peace with the business side of supporting dying populations. The more you, a death doula, can explain what it is you do in your work, how much it costs, and where your services can be provided, the more people will understand how and why they should work with you. Starting off, here is a list of good questions to ask yourself when looking at the area you hope to serve. Once you see what is available in your community, then you can begin to map out how your work will blend with the services already present. It may be that you are the first death doula in your area. Maybe you will reach out to existing hospice organizations or hospitals and establish a working relationship with them. The options for doula work are wide open. As you work to build your death doula practice, begin by considering these questions:

- Are there already death doulas or even birth doulas practicing in your area?

- Are you planning to support your friends and family, or do you want to serve the members of your community?

- Are you interested in supporting pet death instead of human loss or in addition to it? If yes, are there veterinary clinics in your community?

- Do you want to be paid for your services, or do you want to volunteer your services?

- Does your town or city have any hospice providers, nursing homes, hospitals, retirement communities, funeral homes, mortuaries, or other medical facilities?

- Do you want to start your own practice or partner with an existing business?

- What other services do you provide? (Are you a massage therapist, a nurse, a celebrant, a funeral director, a sound therapist, an energy practitioner, an art therapist, a psychic medium, a counselor, a social worker, a chaplain, etc.?)

- In what ways can you share your work as a death doula with your community to increase awareness of the support you provide?

TAKING PAYMENT FOR YOUR WORK

Another essential part of owning and fully embracing your work as a death doula is to have a plan for how you will receive payment. It is often hard for people who work in nontraditional human service fields to be comfortable with accepting money from the people that they care for. How can you be comfortable with taking money from a dying person? One way is to think of receiving payment as an energy exchange. Money is the physical representation of energy that we trade with to receive goods and services. There is nothing inherently bad about being paid for your work. If you are not able to pay your bills, feed yourself, and care for your life, then you will not be able to be fully present for those that your work serves. Some practicing doulas and therapists work on a sliding scale, which means that the clients pay what they can based on their income. There are other options to taking money, though. Instead of working for payment, you can volunteer. You can also accept payment in trade for items or services that you need. If you choose to volunteer for a business such as a hospice group, hospital, or church, then you do not have to figure out how to take money for your time. You will need to decide if you are willing to accept gifts from the people you support, though.

What is most important here is for you to own that the time and energy that you invest in your work is valuable and is worth something. That something does not have to be money, but it can be. How you handle the payment side of the support you provide to people, whether you volunteer your services or request payment, and the population that you serve is up to you. You will need the same thing that you do for your clients for yourself, make decisions based on what fits best for you and the experience you hope to have.

OWNING THE IMPACT

> *"Hospicing the end of one culture while we midwife the birth of another."*
>
> — JOANNA MACY

By working as a death doula, you will effectively help to create and implement a new model of care for dying people and the communities that surround them. You will be providing soul medicine that takes into account the bigger picture of a person's dying journey and is aware that in some ways, there is more than we can understand in the dying process. You will live with the mystery of it all and help others to live without needing to have a clear answer to every question. You will sit firmly in the awareness that your work will help people let go and acknowledge what is no longer true of their lives while you provide a safe container for them to live what it is that they are experiencing.

The work of a death doula is hard. Awareness, understanding, and acceptance by a dying person and their surrounding circle do not make the actual death any less shocking. The part you play as a guide and supporter of this journey allows the soul time and space to navigate each stage of the dying process – for the dying person, their family and friends, and you.

The wonderful thing about working in the death trades is that as experts study death and begin to integrate the information they find; they take their theoretical testing, spiritual studies, life experiences, further learning, and add it to the models of supporting dying people. Working as a death doula means you are allowed to weave models and ideas from many thought areas – scientific, spiritual, real-world experience – into your work. This is how science works, but I just call it life. Do this in your own practice as a death doula. Take your education, any training you have gone through, add your lived experiences, your beliefs, and the knowledge you gain through doing your work, and begin to assemble and distill your own version of the models that work for you.

10

YOU ARE YOUR FIRST CLIENT

"Our fear of death enslaves us to the illusion that we will live forever."

— TERRY TEMPEST WILLIAMS

What else do you need to know about the process of guiding the dying as a death doula? Assuming that you do not have a life-limiting illness, you do not know how it feels to answer the questions we put in front of the people we support for yourself and your life. Although we can never fully know how we will experience our dying time, we can give our clients the dignity of facing the questions we ask them.

This part of the book will lead you through the steps of putting yourself in the dying's shoes. Maybe you have experience with this. Maybe you have your medical and legal paperwork in order. That is good, but it does not eliminate the need for this type of self-examination because although in your work you will be serving others, you must first serve yourself. Holocaust survivor and therapist Dr. Edith Eger says that we can't take people further than we have been ourselves. While I am not asking you to die, I am asking you to sit and contemplate the values and wishes you want to live at the end of your life because dying is something that you will live through too.

WHERE TO BEGIN

You will begin your journey of being a death doula by walking yourself through the same steps that you will walk with your clients. This chapter will guide you on how to plan for your own end of life by building a map of your deathbed ecosystem, completing your end-of-life paperwork, and working your way through all the client questions throughout the book to identify your end-of-life priorities and life values.

Doing this now, in advance, benefits you two-fold. First, you are not under the pressure of knowing your death is coming soon, so you can answer the questions with less pressure. Second, because you are not in your dying time, you have time to make changes to your plans later after you complete them.

The easiest place to start is with what is outside of your body – the paperwork. One of the biggest limiting factors in completing end-of-life paperwork is ensuring that the documents are witnessed or notarized. So, before you begin your paperwork, identify who will be your witnesses or where you will get it notarized. You will want multiple copies of any medical end-of-life documents to add to your chart with your primary health provider, one for safekeeping for yourself and one for whomever you designate to be a surrogate. This also applies to legal documents, one copy for your lawyer, one for yourself, and one for the person you chose to act on your behalf. In this chapter and at the back of the book you will find a link to an overview of what legal and medical paperwork is available for end-of-life planning. In it, you will also find other end-of-life terminology and considerations to make when working on the business side of your life. Use this as a guide to identify what documents you should complete and what information such as passwords and accounts that should be organized to best serve those who would be left behind in the event of your death.

It is important to note here, that the information this book provides is not a substitute for speaking with your personal doctors and lawyers. It is meant as a starting point to empower you to complete your end-of-life documents. If you have any medical conditions that would warrant support from your primary medical provider in making decisions, then schedule an appointment to talk through your end-of-life planning. If your provider will not help you, find someone who will. The same applies to legal matters. If you have a complex financial situation with various assets or have dependents, find a lawyer that specializes in walking you through the process. There are resources online available to assist you in this process like the Five Wishes document or other legal services. Check to make sure that any documents you create online are legal in your region.

Another limiting factor in executing this part of end-of-life planning is talking with the people you pick to be your healthcare agents or legal power of attorney. The people you choose need to be consulted, and they should agree to do this for you. Some people may not agree to do this. Some people may not want to have the discussion. That may be a sign that they are not the right person for the job. Now that you have learned tools and techniques for having complicated conversations, this part may go smoother. If anything, the act of having these conversations with the people in your own life will provide you with practice for when you begin serving people in their dying time.

Add to medical and legal documents any life insurance policies that you have and any funeral planning that you have completed. As far as funeral planning goes, you should have an idea of what type of ceremony you would like to have or if you do not want one at all. What I have heard from many people that I have worked with is that they do not want any ceremony after they die to be sad. I push back on people when I hear this and ask them, "If you lose something that you love or are deeply connected to, do you not think you'll feel sad?" Sadness and grief go hand in hand with the things that we have strong attachments to. I encourage you to arrange for fun, party-like death ceremonies if that is what you want to have, but do not discourage those you leave behind from being sad. Allow them to feel what they feel and do not take away their connection to their own emotions.

If what you plan requires specific paperwork – for example, donating your body to a scientific organization – make sure that is completed, too. Add your disposition forms to your other end-of-life papers and communicate your wishes with the people who need to know.

Part of your end-of-life plans may include building a legacy for the people that you leave behind. If you are not aware of your imminent death, then you have more time to create this. I know a healthy woman in her forties who writes letters to her teenage children every year on their birthday to be given to them later in life. You do not have to be actively dying to actively work on the legacy you will leave behind. The legacy that you leave behind begins with what you start building today.

As far as the business of your life, feel free to collect your accounts and passwords in one place. I recommend this being done digitally in some type of digital vault, a secure online platform that collects and stores digital assets, like Dashlane, Everplans, Cake, GoodTrust, etc. instead of on paper, but feel free to work with what you are comfortable. Depending on the type of digital vault used, a wider range of information can be archived.

Now that you have completed a good portion of the practical side of end-of-life planning – which you may need a lot more than what was described earlier in the chapter – you can begin to get into the deeper part of the work.

To do this first, I recommend that you revisit the death doula reflection client questions throughout the book and answer the questions for yourself. Answering the questions may be tough as they ask you reflect on your own dying time. The skills and practices that you will use with the people that you serve will be first used to support yourself while you find the answers to the questions. Allow yourself to be open to the thoughts and emotions that come up, give them time and a place to be acknowledged and felt. Practice nonjudgement and respond to thoughts and ideas as though you would as if you were speaking to a friend and they answered the same way. We often speak to other people with more kindness when they are talking about difficult topics than we do ourselves. Start exercising your kindness muscle by being kind to yourself. Give yourself some time to think about what quality means for you. What essence of home do you want to be surrounded by in your dying time? Who do you want to be present with you? What comforts you? This can all be completed by answering the same questions that you may pose to the people you serve. After all, it is difficult to take care of others if you are not properly taking care of yourself.

The last thing to do is share what you have decided with important people in your life. This will not only help you because they will have an idea of what your wishes are, but it will also give them permission to begin thinking about this for themselves. By completing this work for yourself, you will be feeding the relationships that will be left behind when your dying time comes.

STEPS FOR IDENTIFYING WISHES FOR A WELL-MANAGED DEATH

Complete these steps based on your current age and life status. Once you completed the steps for your current age, it is fine to go back and consider what your wishes would be at a future age.

1. Paperwork, paperwork, paperwork

    a. Go to https://www.rubyhanson.com/businesofdying and familiarize yourself with the available medical and legal paperwork. Choose what fits with your life and situation best and complete. Also, review the list of recommended information to gather concerning your daily living. Create your business of daily living list.

2. Build Your Deathbed Ecosystem

    a. Go back and answer client questions in the death doula reflection sections to identify your wishes and areas that you may need to work on before your dying time.

3. Important practical information to identify:

    a. Who will you name to be your healthcare agent/ power of attorney?

b. Where would you like to be in your dying time?

c. What rituals or ceremonies would you like before/ after death?

d. Where is your end-of-life paperwork?

e. Funeral arrangements/ body disposition wishes

4. Review your finances and insurance policies to ensure that your wishes are financially possible. If additional financial support is needed, begin researching what is available in your community, what social service support is offered, and what the qualifying requirements are.

5. Last, have the courageous conversations with the people in your life concerning your end-of-life wishes.

INCREASE YOUR ABILITY TO NOTICE

While you are working on your end-of-life paperwork, you can begin to utilize some of the techniques you learned throughout this book on yourself. In this chapter, you will find more tools that will support your own personal being as you begin death doula work with yourself as your first client.

Environmental Awareness Exercise

This exercise's purpose is to start to build your awareness of your surroundings and tap into your physical and emotional state of being. Working on these skills will help you to interact in the deathbed room by actively noticing the environment around you. What you feel in the space may be being felt by others, the dying person, and those attending to them. This practice can help you develop your ability to "read the field."

This exercise can be done sitting or standing. It can even be done while moving around unless you prefer to do it with your eyes closed. In that case, take a seat and get comfortable. Begin by recalling a scene outside. Where are you? What is the weather like? Describe to yourself what you are seeing with your eyes. How does it feel on your skin? Think about how the weather can be noticed by your different physical senses. Can you smell anything? What do you hear? What does the temperature feel like? What words go along with these sensations? Where do you notice your body? What emotions come up during this experience? Go ahead and release this practice. Feel free to write in a journal what you noticed.

The next part of this practice is to access different sensations as you have experienced them or how you would imagine them to be.

Imagine yourself in a building. You step outside and instantly you sense that it is going to snow. What do you notice…

With your eyes?

With your ears?

What do you smell?

How does your skin feel?

Describe where your body is.

Describe what you think about the fact that is going to snow.

Describe how you feel about the upcoming snow.

Can you tell what direction the storm is coming from?

Put words to anything else that comes to your mind.

Now, let's do this again, but this time, imagine that you are on a ride at the fair or at a theme park.

What do you notice…

With your eyes?

With your ears?

What do you smell?

How does your skin feel?

Describe where your body is.

Describe what you think about the fact that you are on this ride.

Describe how you feel about the ride.

Put words to anything else that comes to your mind.

Both of these exercises are designed to help you begin to deepen your understanding of how you use your senses to interpret your world. Every day, we move around in our environment noticing things. Many times, the way we notice our surroundings is limited. We have been taught that our ability to experience the world around is limited to five senses when, in fact, we have more senses. Our expanded senses include our sense of hearing, sight, taste, touch, smell along with:

- Equilibrioception – a sense of balance. This is what keeps us upright and helps us make our way around without getting hurt.

- Proprioception – knowing which parts of your body are where without looking. It's how we can type without looking at the keyboard, for instance, or walk around without having to watch our feet.

- Kinaesthesia – sense of movement.

- Thermoception – we know whether our environment is too cold or too hot. Being able to sense the temperature around us helps keep us alive and well.

- Nociception – the ability to feel pain.

- Chronoception – how we sense the passing of time.

It is helpful to be knowledgeable when it comes to the broader range of human senses when working with dying people because the dying process can interfere with, disrupt, and modify the way people experience the world. These sensory changes can affect the way people interact in their deathbed ecosystem. The educated death doula can watch for changes in these areas as indications of how a person is progressing through their dying journey.

Your skills as a death doula will improve through walking yourself through the end-of-life planning stages and by increasing your ability to be a noticer in your environment. The completion of your own plans will better prepare you for the hard work of serving others in their dying time. Realistically, you may not implement everything you learn in this book in your practice as a death doula, but all the material presented and all the prework that you have completed prior to working with anyone will help to be a more well-rounded doula and person.

It is essential to not only know how to fully support other people as they journey through the dying process, but you also need to have tools and techniques for how to maintain your personal being in order to continue functioning as a death doula.

PREPARING YOURSELF FOR SUPPORTING DEATH

What you bring into the dying space within your body is more important than what you fill your doula bag with. There needs to be concentrated time and effort poured into your own being in order to be able to fully serve another person in their dying time. This learning portion covers boundary creation, grounding, balancing, and releasing practices that will support you in your ability to work as a death doula for many years to come. Death doulas also need to be able to spend time reflecting on their own experiences and what they see reflected of themselves in the people that they serve. The topics discussed next will help you as the death doula deepen your sense of presence by connecting to yourself and establishing healthy habits for interacting with others whether they are in the dying space or not.

Boundaries

Working with other people means that death doulas will be working with others' emotions. It is important that doulas provide support for people's emotions while not owning them permanently. It is essential that death doulas be able to identify and verbalize what other people are experiencing, their emotions around it, and how it is influencing the environment around them. There need to be healthy boundaries set up to deal with how doulas take on other people's emotional experiences. There also need to be boundaries that protect the doula's energy and ability to perform their tasks. There will be times when the line between what is being experienced by those in the deathbed ecosystem and the doula will be thin, and that is okay. It is the job of the doula to fully dive into the moment in order to serve their people, but there can come a time when the death doula carries too much and may not be able to let go of it all. That is when problems can arise.

First, let's identify types of boundaries and what they mean for the death doula. Loose boundaries mean that the doula is catching other people's pain. It shows up as mirroring other people's emotions, taking on too much responsibility, or getting sick. Loose boundaries are okay for interpreting what is being felt by those in the deathbed space. It is good to know what physical and emotional manifestations are occurring in the space without speaking about them. It can become too much though if what is being taken on by the death doula cannot be released and overshadows their own internal experience.

Firm boundaries are exactly opposite of loose in that they do not allow for using intuition and inner wisdom to understand what people in the deathbed space are experiencing due to being walled off. This can show up as frustration, anger, acting uncaring, or being tense. It is in this space that a person can dehumanize another and treat them poorly.

Balanced boundaries allow the death doula to be in touch with their own feeling and sense of self and the others. Being in balance and having established boundaries means that what the death doula takes on from the other does not feel like a burden. The emotions and physical experiences do not have to come home with the doula, meaning the support provided will not prevent the doula from getting a good night's rest on a regular basis.

With time and experience, as a practicing death doula, you will learn what boundaries you need to put in place in order to fully serve your clients and to remain healthy and active in your own life.

Grounding

To be present for the entirety of another person's being, the death doula must have a firm connection to who they are in their core being. What happens in the dying space can figuratively knock people off their feet. Grounding practices bring a person back to who they are and allow them to handle complex situations and emotions like those that occur in a person's dying time. Engaging in a grounding exercise can also be a good practice for a doula to do before entering a deathbed ecosystem because it allows the person to set aside what is happening in their own life outside of the space and focus their energy on the work ahead. This ability to ground yourself empowers any other practice you provide to the dying. Grounding assists caregivers when their energy is depleted or unsettled. Before you massage or attempt any hands-on therapy, therefore, you need to balance your own energy using this exercise. Otherwise, you will simply be passing on your anxiety to the dying person. You can practice it on your own or use the instructions to guide the dying person or those in the circle around them.

Like a Tree

An ancient Chinese internal energy exercise (Chi Kung) known as "Standing Like a Tree" is excellent for calming the entire nervous system. It is normally done standing, but it can be done while sitting. The stationary positions promote increased circulation and deeper breathing and induce inner calm.

1. Simply stand or sit with your feet shoulder-width apart. Unlock your knees slightly. Let your arms rest effortlessly by your sides. Relax your shoulders. Breathe naturally. Slightly lower your gaze or close your eyes. Try remaining quietly in this position for a minute or two to begin with and gradually build up to several minutes if possible.

2. As you are in this position, imagine that your feet are like the roots of a great tree sinking down into the earth. Your body remains unmoving like the trunk of the tree. You imagine that the very top of your head is lightly suspended

from a golden cord reaching up infinitely into the sky; it is as if your head was as relaxed as the countless leaves of the tree opening into the sunlight.

Variation on this exercise if you are in bed:

Lie flat with your legs slightly separated. Flex your feet so that your toes are nearly at right angles to your legs. Imagine you are holding a large balloon in your arms, over your stomach. Try to stay in that position for a short while, relax and repeat whenever you wish.

Balancing Your Energy

1. Sit comfortably, trying, if possible, to keep your back straight. Rest your feet flat on the floor.

2. Close your eyes or lower your gaze.

3. Relax your shoulders and chest and breathe naturally.

4. Bring your mind to bear on the fact that you are sitting. Try to feel the weight of your entire upper body resting on your sitting bones and the bones themselves feeling the pressure of that weight. Focus your awareness on the bottom of your spine. Try to feel the strength of the base of your spine as it supports the full weight of your spinal cord and skull.

5. As you become more aware of the sense of strength at the base of your spine, allow your neck, shoulders, and chest to relax further as if they were allowing the spine to bear their weight fully.

6. Then, without losing that feeling, let your mind also be aware of the very top of your head. Imagine your head being very gently supported as if suspended from above by a fine cord.

7. Then let your attention move slowly down from the top of your head, down your neck, and slowly down your backbone. Imagine each of the vertebrae in your neck and back, and as you call each one to mind, imagine it is relaxing and becoming warm. It is almost as if a warm current were starting to travel from the top of your spine slowly down to the very bottom.

Releasing

In order to function as a death doula, a person needs to have an active practice for releasing all that they see and take on when working in the death trade. This will allow not only for the person to step fully into their own life outside of their work, but it will also create boundaries by having rituals that signal to the body and inner being what energy, physical sensations, and emotions are yours to keep and what belongs to the other person. It does not have to be a complex ritual. Releasing can include the practice of taking a bath, watching a certain show, having a particular tea, pressure point massage, therapeutic tremoring (shaking), or doing a specific breathing exercise. When and where it takes place depends on the person and what works for them. Finding what works best for you may take some trial and error. It also may change depending on the experience you are trying to release.

Letting go or releasing what is taken on in the dying space does not mean that the death doula never thinks about the experience again. What it does is create a healthy separation from what took place in the dying space and what goes on in the individual Doula's life.

Release Exercise:

Take a couple of deep breaths. Begin to center yourself in the moment. Say the following statement out loud:

I command that all the energies and emotions that do not belong to me be immediately sent back to their original source, never to return again, now.

Now that you have covered most of what is needed to begin working as a death doula and you feel that this is a way that you can serve others, you must face the reasons that might prevent you from taking on any clients. In the next chapter, we will discuss why you should reconsider working as a death doula. Even though the work is rewarding, it is full of pitfalls and reasons why you may want to run for the hills before ever working with one dying person.

11

WHY YOU SHOULD NOT BE A DEATH DOULA

Let's be frank. Being a death doula is not for everyone. You might even be thinking that all the information in the book is great and everything, but working as a death doula is not something that you think you can actually do. Currently, very few people know what a death doula is. How can you possibly help people when they do not know your job exists? Who in their right mind really wants to talk about death? The people who are willing to talk to you about their deaths are going to want concrete answers, but you may not have clear-cut responses to their questions. The work might be stressful and sad and may not happen in a regularly scheduled manner. And ultimately, it is working with death. People might think that you are weird, strange, or morbid for doing this kind of work. Plus, how can you ask people to pay for this type of support? It feels like you are taking advantage of them.

In some aspects, all the thoughts listed in the previous paragraph might pop into your head at some point, and all of them are valid.

WHAT IS IT THAT YOU DO AGAIN?

Up until the late 1960s hospice did not exist. It was not until Dame Cicely Saunders decided that she wanted to improve the conditions for dying people in Britain that the hospice model of care was born. Now, the concept of hospice is a common one with 1.55 million people entering into its care in 2018, according to the National Hospice and Palliative Care Organization. While hesitancy still may exist among the public to enter into hospice care, its use is increasing yearly. And when people finally experience the level of care provided by someone trained to support the dying, they often ask why they did not decide to do it sooner. The same thoughts that go for why people did not think to start using hospice care sooner apply to working with a death doula. Once someone starts doing the work of facing their death with someone who is trained to make the experience one full of growth and deep connection, they wonder why they did not undertake it sooner.

One of the main roles I take on as a death doula is to be a death educator. I feel that it is my job to share the options available to people in their dying time. This occurs often in my daily exchanges with people. What is funniest about this is my friends, acquaintances, and even family will engage in deep conversations about end-of-life planning with me and still say, "Now what is it that you do?" I respond, "The conversation we just had is a big part of what I do." I have been told that there is no such thing as a death doula. My thought on that one is I wonder if the people who train and employ death doulas know that. I had no idea that I did not exist. I have even been told that the name death doula itself is off-putting to people. Yep. People who are not turned away by the word "death" can be left confused by the "doula." I get it. It is not a phrase that many use, and when they do, it is often to reference a birth doula. My friend Beth Krom came up with a way to describe what a death doula does to those who are left confused by the title. Her acronym is:

D – Demystifying
O – Our
U – Understanding of
L – Life
A – And Death

Her description is spot-on in describing part of what a death doula does. Through our work helping others plan for and come to terms with the dying process, in our work in bringing sacredness back to the dying process, we help people learn to live openly and fully in their present life, no matter their current physical state of being. And that is healing for everyone, not just the dying.

THE INEVITABLE TOLL

For all of the feel-good ideas that come along with the idea of being a death doula, the work does take a toll. If not managed properly, your physical being may not endure the process of serving multiple people in their dying. The work of a death doula can be physically tiring, emotionally demanding, spiritually and mentally challenging, but it is also rewarding to know that you are serving people in one of their most vulnerable times. Birth doulas help women to bring babies into the world from darkness to light. Death doulas help guide people out of the world of light into darkness. Both experiences are transformative. Some people even say in birth we are taken from the world of spirit into the physical world, and in death, we are taken from the physical world back into the world of spirit. It can be intense work in its beauty and in its sadness.

The range of experiences had by death doulas are vast.

There are people in this world who are willing to and who are seeking out people with whom they can talk openly about their dying time. In our culture, that kind of talk is usually rushed along or pushed aside because it can be uncomfortable to have those conversations. As a death doula, you give the people permission to talk about their worries related to death, their wishes for their dying time, and how they will be remembered after their death. Your work allows them to live in spite of dying.

Working in the death trade does not make you weird or morbid. It does not make you any less of a human than someone who works in an office every day for a living. You know what is weird? Living a life pretending that people do not die. Westernized cultures are pretty skilled at doing just that: closeting away death and talking about it very little. It does not serve us as humans to not acknowledge that our life is limited. No, you do not have to go around reminding everyone of that fact every day of your life unless you want to. As a death doula, you are not even required to engage in conversations about dying every day. But you may find that you develop such strength and groundedness in the fact that everything must die at some point that people will seek you out without even knowing why they are doing so to talk about these things.

There was a point in time when working with a therapist was not common practice. For some, it is still not acceptable, but working on mental health has become prevalent, and the type of professionals available to work with has grown. I like to think that working on end-of-life matters and bringing back sacredness to the dying process is following the same pattern. The work that a death doula does is needed, and the opportunity to provide care will only increase for those who are trained in the art of being a death doula.

I CAN'T TAKE PAYMENT FOR THIS

One major hurdle in working with dying populations is taking payment. How you will be able to take money from people for the services you provide depends on you and your relationship with money. It has helped me immensely to think of money as an energy exchange. Money is the physical manifestation of energy. We use our bodies and mind to work, and in trade, we are given money. That is how our monetary system is set up. It helps to group the death doulas work with that of a therapist or a life coach. People pay for those services. What the doula provides is valuable and worthy of charging money for. Another option is for the death doula to work as a volunteer. Plenty of hospices, churches, nursing homes, and hospitals use volunteer services to support the people in the communities they serve. Neither option is the better choice. It is what is right for you and the people you are working with.

WHAT IF I DON'T KNOW THE ANSWER?

As far as having all the answers for the questions that people ask about death dying, you will not have all the answers. Life is not built that way. The measure of control that we are sure that we have in our daily lives is a thin veil. None knows for sure how long we have to live in our bodies. None of us can guarantee what the next day will bring. We have confidence that we can, but that confidence is surrendered when faced with grave events like during a pandemic or a natural disaster or when diagnosed with a terminal illness or as we grow older.

You will have nights after working as a death doula when you will go to bed angry, sad, confused, or all three. Questions will remain, but the one answer that will be clear is that you were there for someone. You did not allow your discomfort or unease to prevent you from being present and fully witnessing and supporting another person's dying journey, and that is a gift.

As a practicing death doula, no matter if you are paid for your work or volunteer your services, no matter if you support only your family and friends or you serve the greater community around you, your work has worth. Your work is necessary. Your work makes the world around you a better place by serving others. The time and efforts you invest in death doula work will help people make decisions about their end of life that will guide them so that they are able to focus on spending their last moments in ways that align with their truest self.

PROTECTING AND PRESERVING YOUR PERSONAL BEING

Being a death doula is intense, albeit rewarding work. It can be full of your own emotions and other people's reactions to the events unfolding. The work can also be physically exhausting. Just like giving birth, dying knows no schedule. You may often find yourself at people's bedside at all hours of the night.

In order to be effective in your work as a death doula, you must take care of yourself. How can you properly support a person during their death journey if you are not taking care of yourself? "If Society wants us to keep caring for others, it's going to have to show a little more care for us," says Kate Washington, author of *Already Toast: Caregiving and Burnout in America* says. A starting point in knowing how your body is functioning and whether or not it needs something to keep going is key to understanding what your normal looks like. Many of us push past what is healthy for ourselves by working when ill, not resting, or by eating whatever is within reach. Many more of us do not realize that our bodies are not functioning at the best of their ability. It is easy to lean on the self-care and maintenance of getting enough sleep, eating well, and exercising but there is more to self-care than that. Recognizing and admitting what the internal relationship we have with our physical bodies looks like and how we mentally interact with ourselves can be challenging. Self-care is more complicated than diet or exercise.

> *"Endless caregiving, especially in isolation, has a negative impact on the caregivers' health. They can raise blood pressure, disrupt sleep, and trigger anxiety and depression."*
>
> — L.S. DUGDALE

In order to become a more skilled noticer, just like using your own body to frame what all is within the realm of the physical human experience, death doulas can access their own mental and emotional interactions with themselves and with others to grow skills of observation. By increasing our ability to notice what is going on in our own experience, we can begin to more keenly observe others.

Once we identify that our own person needs care and kindness in order to work at the level necessary to serve others, we can begin to engage in practices that refill our own reserves. And by filling our own reserves, we are better able to be fully present with those who are dying.

DEATH DOULA STARTER PACK

Why do you want to work as a death doula?

Are you prepared to handle the intensity that comes along with the work?

How are you currently taking care of yourself?

How well do you know your body?

How well do you know your mind?

Are you your own friend?

What are your body's discrete/ small responses to intense emotions?

What are your body's big responses to intense emotions?

Do you know what it looks like when your mind or body needs a break?

Self-Soothing Exercise

(Adapted from the Center for Mindful Self-Compassion)

The intention of this exercise is to identify what physical comfort, which you can provide to yourself, looks like. It is valuable to tune into the small movements and gestures that we do in times of stress, when relaxing enough to fall asleep, when supporting another whether it be in past jobs or comforting a small child. We will access the experiences you have already lived to identify what works for you and find opportunities to add self-soothing into your daily life whenever you need to access it. I call it covert comfort when I teach it to people who need to use it in a stressful work situation or to children feeling stress in an environment when they do not want attention brought to their emotional or physical discomfort. Once a person begins to practice this exercise with themselves, they can begin to notice other ways that people provide comfort to themselves. A word of caution: this practice is not intended to teach people how to cover up or mask their physical and emotional discomforts. It is taught with the idea of awareness. Once we allow ourselves to be aware of what we are experiencing and identify what emotion or sensation it is, we can begin to understand it and why it is there.

To begin, sit in a comfortable position. You can lie down if preferred. Now, begin to ask yourself, what feels genuinely supportive to me?

Bring your palms of your hands together.

Take a couple of deep breaths

How do they feel? Start to gently rub them back and forth. What do you feel? Heat? Friction? Maybe you notice that your hands are dry.

Next, move your hands into a cupped position. Feel free to rest them in your lap.

Breathe in and out. Allow yourself to feel the openness of your hands. Allow yourself to feel open to this practice.

Take both of your hands and place them on your heart region.

What feeling is there?

Breathe in and out.

Now, you can begin to circle one hand on your chest.

Remember to breathe.

Give yourself permission to notice how this movement feels to you.

Now, I want you to keep one hand on your heart and place the other hand on your belly.

Our bellies are a place where we hold a lot of expectations. Just allow your belly to relax. No need to hold it in or keep it tight.

Take a deep breath.

Move your second hand onto your belly. Let yourself relax further.

What do you notice?

Now, bring one of your hands up and place it on your cheek. How does it feel? Notice it without judgment.

Breathe deeply.

Place your two hands on your cheeks. Often, we do this motion when we think something is precious.

Place one of your hands on your forehead. What are you feeling?

Breath in and out.

Now I want you to cross your arms over your chest and hug yourself.

Remember to breathe.

Move your hug up to your shoulders. Gently squeeze them.

Next, move your hug down to your belly. Squeeze gently.

Breathe in and out.

Release your belly and stroke one of your forearms.

Now, bring your hands back together and take a few more deep breaths.

This is the part of the exercise where I invite you to explore on your own.

One of the best ways to explain self-soothing movements and gestures is to talk about holding a baby. What do most people do when you place a baby in their arms? They rock to comfort the baby, but have you ever sat in a room where one person is rocking while holding a baby and witnessed other people in the room begin to rock too? Using self-soothing movements and gestures are essentially habits. It is good to recognize what habits you use currently in your life and then add to them as needed.

To finish up this practice, I usually tell people the story about my mom and one of the ways she would comfort herself that drove me absolutely nuts when I was a kid. I saw her doing this mostly when she was relaxed, sitting on the couch watching T.V. Why this drove me nuts? Who knows. She would tuck one of her hands palm-down on her collarbone, tips of her hand inside her shirt. The funniest part of this is that I use this same gesture all the time.

The ways we soothe ourselves in one situation may not work for another. Tucking my hand into my shirt collar is not how I would want to support myself during a business meeting in a conference room. Instead, I provide other means to fidget or connect with my physical self by wearing bracelets that I can touch or rings that I can twirl. What works for the individual is personal and dependent on their starting point. Not everyone has the same physical ability level. Not everyone likes touch, even their own.

12

YOUR WORK'S IMPACT

"What does all this work mean? That is for you to decide. It has to be your answer, from the deepest part of your heart, or else you won't be able to continue in your work."

— L.S. DUGDALE

I wrote this book because I wanted to change the way we deal with and understand death and the process of dying. Like I mentioned earlier in Chapter 10, if things work out as they should, I will be gone when it is my children's time to die. I will not be here to support them physically, emotionally, and spiritually and fill their last days on this planet with comfort, contentment, and ease. So to ensure that they receive that kind of care, I started training people to create a world that would support them. By training others, I am creating a new model of supporting dying people. It blends our allopathic western medicine with the skills and gifts we already carry inside of us. It is but one drop of water in the ocean that ripples out and touches much more than just one reader. You are my drop in the ocean.

Becoming a death doula allowed me to pull all my life experiences with death and dying and give myself space and time to heal my own journey. As a healthcare worker, I did not receive much support from the facilities that I worked at when patients died. I was surprised by how other people on my team reacted when we lost patients. Many of my coworkers did not know how to handle the death of a patient. Culturally, we have been conditioned to push death and dying away and not talk about it. We have been conditioned to not speak of it even when it is happening to someone we love, someone we are working on, and even ourselves. It is my biggest hope that this book will allow people to once again begin to openly discuss death and develop some skills to support people when their time comes in order to better prepare the world for their own deaths that blends the methods used in allopathic medicine with deeper soul medicine. And that starts with healing your own personal experiences and owning your ability to support others in their dying time. If you read this book and help many people or only one person in their dying time, then my work has been a success.

My philosophy is that we learn how to die by watching others die. How can we do that if we never see or talk about dying? In this book, you have learned skills to start those conversations. If you can carry away one message from my writing it should be that you were equipped from the moment you were born to do this work. All you need is already within you. Your willingness to work with the dying is the biggest hurdle to overcome in training to be a death doula because not everyone wants to walk this path and not everyone should. All of the other learning is just skills to identify and polish up. Being a death doula looks different for every person. It is up to you to decide how it will look for you.

Life is not a race that anyone is going to win. If we allow ourselves to embrace the fear, anger, uncertainty, and all the complex emotions that surface when someone is faced with a terminal diagnosis or when someone dies unexpectedly, we allow room for growing through that experience. We make room for the fullness of a holistic death. You can help provide that. Your ability to empower someone to die a holistic death includes not only what happens to their physical bodies, but what happens to their inner self, their emotional states, the world and legacy that they leave behind; it also allows them to teach our people how to carry their being forward in life when their physical selves are no longer present.

Give yourself permission to see how far and deep you will go into the subject that you may already have had much experience with. Who can say how the process will open up your perspective even more to what is possible when we as a culture begin to allow space for the idea that our time in our physical bodies is limited and valuable? That thought process gives permission to be willing to try new things and to reach out to people who have a desire to enrich their lives in this area. By learning about death, you will be able to live more deeply in the present time. You will be able to embrace the experienced knowledge that you have gained through work and family experiences. You will also be equipped to have conversations with people when they are in one of their most vulnerable times.

To read, write, and live the idea of the impermanence of our existence allows for deeper connections with others because this work allows us to cut through the small talk and reach out to people where they need healing most. Another thing that happened in writing this book was the community that I created by opening myself up to the idea that I have something of value to share with others. That has not only been important for my own life, but it also taught me that this is something that people who are dying wrestle with. Have their lives contributed something of value to others? How will they be remembered? What will people say about them when they are gone? These are questions that I identified that the dying person must be allowed to ask in order to fully embrace the end of their life. These are also questions that those sitting with dying people must not rush to answer. The process of writing this book and companioning with dying populations is not that dissimilar. In both instances, we think we know what is going to happen; we can recognize the fear that comes up. Am I enough? Did I say enough? How can I connect with those that are with me now? Will this process hurt? What happens when what I thought was going to happen never comes true? What do I do with all that I do not know?

If anything, being a death doula teaches us that we have to surrender to the ideas, thoughts, and experiences we have surrounding death and dying because, for as much as we think we know, we really know very little. All the prep work and learning can help you to be open to what will happen when you are present with a dying person, but it makes no guarantees about how the process will go. And that is what is beautiful about the work you will do and the soul care that you will provide. You will be the safe container for people to experience death. Your presence, your skills, your comfort with uncertainty will model to all those surrounding the dying how we can create a new and improved model of caring and supporting those in their dying time.

What we do in life, we do in death. We are led to believe that death is a time of loss – loss of control, loss of body, loss of relationship – but much is unknown in life and out of our control.

The illusion lies in our idea that life is full of certainty and death is full of uncertainty when, in fact, they are both the same.

So, where does this leave you? Hopefully, more confident and courageous in your ability to support others in their dying time.

ACKNOWLEDGMENTS

Writing a book seems like it would be a solitary process when, in fact, it is not. Although I did most of my typing in the library of my house by myself, my work on this book would not have been possible without all of the teachers that came before me.

First, I would like to thank all the people in my life that showed up and unwittingly played the part of a teacher. The many nurses, doctors, surgical techs, housekeepers, and dietary staff at the hospital – the collective experiences and knowledge that you shared with me have made me who I am today. I carry pieces of the lessons you taught me always. To the many patients that I have helped care for over the years at the hospital – what you taught me is hard to find in books or in the classroom. I have held your hands, swabbed your bleeding wounds, wiped your tears, and sometimes helped to make you better, but you have touched my soul. Your trust in the teams that I was on reinforced the idea that I can do difficult things and make a difference. Your vulnerability never allowed me to hide away from my feelings even when I had to carry on working. And for those patients who did not make it, although I never fully knew you in life, I will never forget you. I carry your deaths with me always.

To my night nurses, you taught me how to care for the patients we lost. You taught me how to clean their bodies, how to make them look warm, uncover their hands so they were ready for holding, and in doing so, how to provide comfort to their loved ones as they visited one last time. To the people that I have served as a death doula, even when you did not want to talk death with me, thank you for showing that this work is needed and valuable. You have shared some of the greatest life lessons with me.

I also want to thank my death doula teachers – Tarron Estes, Jan Booth, Wenda Clinard, Trish Rux, and all my classmates, especially my school partner, Kari Allerton. These people are some of the gentlest humans the world has ever seen. Their support and expertise helped me grow my own death doula skills.

Although I have only read his books, I would like to thank Stephen Jenkinson. His work has been pivotal in stretching my ideas and thoughts on life and death. I hope one day to meet him in person.

To all of my EO forum mates over the years, thank you for helping me learn how to ask more purposeful questions.

Also, many thanks to my teacher Dr. Sarah Kerr. Her approach to teaching is light, easy to follow, and impactful.

This book would not have been possible without my family's support and their ability to leave me alone for long stretches of time. Their willingness to ignore me while I worked on this book did not go unnoticed. Thank you to all of you. My hands and heart are overflowing with love and fun because of the three of you.

I wouldn't be able to complete this book without the team

at The Author Incubator. I am forever grateful that Angela Lauria saw the author in me and encouraged me to see her too. And to my editor, Natasa Smirnov, thank you for your support and calm guidance. You made the process of polishing my writing a delightful task.

I cannot forget to mention the people who started me on the journey to being a death doula, my grandparents, my parents, and my ancestors. The way my grandparents included me in their lives allowed me to get to know the elders in my family and be present in their lives, their illnesses, and their deaths. Even when I did not want to visit my aunt in the nursing home, they took me. I am grateful for that experience now.

To my Aunt Micki who first taught me about loss come too early, I am glad that you were my aunt, and I miss you.

To my dad, his honesty and calm wisdom created the foundation on which I stand on today. I can count on him to have long, science-filled conversations where we talk about our family and interests.

To my mom, who tried to give me everything in life and was unable but succeeded in death. To this day, when I have something heavy in my heart that I need help lifting, she takes it.

My parents' mistakes turned out to be my greatest sources of learning and connection. My love for them knows no bounds.

To my sister, what can I say? She is the person who knows the story of where I come from best and therefore knows what in my life laid the foundation for this work. I cannot thank her or her husband enough for loving and supporting me and for openly receiving my love.

To my ancestors – recent and far-removed who I am still trying to learn more about – thank you for surviving and for passing down your strength and courage. I am winking at you, Anne H.

And lastly, thank you to my Great Aunt Mary Ruby who used to come and sit and chat with me when I waited tables. Remember when you said, "Oh, Kelly, you are a writer." Aunt Mary, it turns out you were right.

ABOUT THE AUTHOR

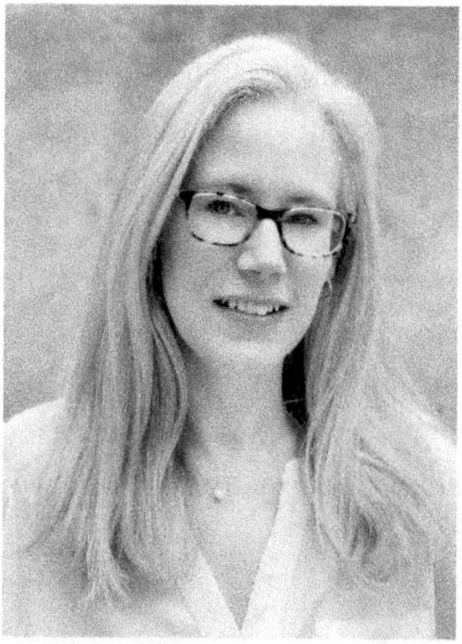

Kelly Ruby Hanson is a Death Doula, certified surgical technologist, and life coach who helps people become death doulas.

Raised in a small farming community where the older generations of her family were close by, Kelly learned what a good death looked like and became an advocate for conscious dying after losing multiple family members as a young adult. After experiencing many deaths in her work at the hospital and then losing her mom, Kelly realized that she needed a different set of skills and tools to better support the losses she and so many others experienced. Kelly learned that to have a better dying experience, people needed more than the traditional medicine could offer. She became certified a death doula through The Conscious Dying Institute to deepen her work with clients.

Now, Kelly combines medical knowledge, practical understanding of the dying process, and conversation skills to teach how to be present with people during their dying time. Her approach blends the language of medicine with holistic practices to develop strength in supporting conscious deaths.

Kelly is a transplant to Colorado. She attended IUPUI where she studied psychology and trained as a surgical technologist at Indiana University Hospital, Methodist, and Riley Hospital.

She loves spending time outdoors, reading, and cooking. She looks back on each death she has supported with gratitude for what it taught her about living life fully and dying openly. She believes every person deserves to die in line with their values, supported by the people who uphold their wishes.

ABOUT DIFFERENCE PRESS

Difference Press is the exclusive publishing arm of The Author Incubator, an educational company for entrepreneurs – including life coaches, healers, consultants, and community leaders – looking for a comprehensive solution to get their books written, published, and promoted. Its founder, Dr. Angela Lauria, has been bringing to life the literary ventures of hundreds of authors-in-transformation since 1994.

A boutique-style self-publishing service for clients of The Author Incubator, Difference Press boasts a fair and easy-to-understand profit structure, low-priced author copies, and author-friendly contract terms. Most importantly, all of our #incubatedauthors maintain ownership of their copyright at all times.

LET'S START A MOVEMENT WITH YOUR MESSAGE

In a market where hundreds of thousands of books are published every year and are never heard from again, The Author Incubator is different. Not only do all Difference

Press books reach Amazon bestseller status, but all of our authors are actively changing lives and making a difference.

Since launching in 2013, we've served over 500 authors who came to us with an idea for a book and were able to write it and get it self-published in less than 6 months. In addition, more than 100 of those books were picked up by traditional publishers and are now available in bookstores. We do this by selecting the highest quality and highest potential applicants for our future programs.

Our program doesn't only teach you how to write a book – our team of coaches, developmental editors, copy editors, art directors, and marketing experts incubate you from having a book idea to being a published, bestselling author, ensuring that the book you create can actually make a difference in the world. Then we give you the training you need to use your book to make the difference in the world, or to create a business out of serving your readers.

ARE YOU READY TO MAKE A DIFFERENCE?

You've seen other people make a difference with a book. Now it's your turn. If you are ready to stop watching and start taking massive action, go to http://theauthorincubator.com/apply/.

"Yes, I'm ready!"

OTHER BOOKS BY DIFFERENCE PRESS

Skinny Genes: The Surprising Truth about Every Body's Capacity to Settle at a Natural Weight, Even When Diets Have Failed by Arianne Bozarth, CNS, MS

Family Business Legacy Plan: The Ultimate Guide to Creating a Legacy for Your Family without Paying too Much in Taxes by Maria L. Ellis, MBA

iMove: Helping Your Clients Heal from Compulsive Exercise by Amy Gardner, MS, CERD, RYT

Rising Beyond Betrayal: One Woman's Guest for Peace after Tragedy, Trauma, and Loss by Lise-Marie Monroe

The Essential Oil Business: A Heart-Centered Entrepreneur's Guide to Adding a New Stream of Revenue by Lori Rothschild, PhD

True Gifts: Ignite Your Soul Magic and Monetize the Highest Expression of Your Purpose by Jewel Veitch

No More Playing Small: Free Your Inner Rockstar and Go All in on Your Full-Time Coaching Career by Megan Jo Wilson

THANK YOU

Thank you for getting this book, which shows your desire to make a difference in people's lives and deaths. Your decision to travel on the path to become a death doula and serve those who are navigating the end of their lives is not one to be taken lightly. The work can be challenging, but it is also rewarding.

Visit https://www.rubyhanson.com/businessofdying for the pdf version of the bonus chapter "The Business of Dying" that covers end-of-life paperwork, death and dying terminology, and a daily living business checklist to use as you guide your clients in their end-of-life planning.

I would love to learn more about your journey and experiences supporting others during their end-of-life transitions. Death doula work is made better when we have the support of a community that understands what it is we do best. Please keep in touch (I'm most active on Facebook at https://www.facebook.com/yourlocaldeathdoula and Instagram @KHansoncoaching) and visit https://www.rubyhanson.com for more resources.

www.ingramcontent.com/pod-product-compliance
Lightning Source LLC
LaVergne TN
LVHW022206200926
848481LV00006B/1871